Immunotherapy of Hepatocellular Carcinoma

Tim F. Greten
Editor

Immunotherapy of Hepatocellular Carcinoma

Springer

Editor
Tim F. Greten
Thoracic and Gastrointestinal Oncology Branch
Center for Cancer Research, National Cancer Institute
Bethesda, MD, USA

ISBN 978-3-319-64957-3 ISBN 978-3-319-64958-0 (eBook)
DOI 10.1007/978-3-319-64958-0

Library of Congress Control Number: 2017953935

Printed on acid-free paper

This Springer imprint is published by Springer Nature
The registered company is Springer International Publishing AG
The registered company address is: Gewerbestrasse 11, 6330 Cham, Switzerland

Preface

Hepatocellular carcinoma (HCC) is the third most common cause of cancer related death in the United States. Treatment options are limited. Viral hepatitis is one of the major risk factors for HCC, which represents a typical "inflammation-induced" cancer.

Immune-based treatment approaches have revolutionized oncology in recent years. Various treatment strategies have received FDA approval including dendritic cell vaccination, for prostate cancer, as well as immune checkpoint inhibition targeting the CTLA4 or the PD1/PDL1 axis in melanoma, lung, and kidney cancer. Additionally, cell-based therapies (adoptive T cell therapy, CAR T cells and TCR transduced T cells) have demonstrated significant efficacy in patients with B cell malignancies and melanoma. Immune checkpoint inhibitors in particular have generated enormous excitement across the entire field of oncology, providing significant benefit to a minority of patients.

In this book we provide insights into liver – cancer and immunology. Experts in the field provide an overview of fundamental immunological questions in liver cancer and tumorimmunology, which form the base for immune-based approaches in HCC, which are gaining increasing interest in the community due to first promising results obtained in early clinical trials.

Bethesda, MD, USA | Tim F. Greten

Contents

Introduction

Every year, more than 800 Mio people die from hepatocellular cancer (HCC) worldwide making HCC one of the deadliest diseases in the world. Standard of care treatment options are limited and very distinct from other types of solid cancer including surgical resection, orthotopic liver transplantation, local ablative therapies, transarterial chemoembolization, and radiation and systemic therapy with TKIs. More than 80% of patients with HCC have different types of underlying liver diseases causing possible liver dysfunction making treatment of this disease much difficult. Despite efforts from basic scientist, clinical investigators, biotech companies, and biopharma, very little progress has been made in the past 10 years. However, this may change with the advent of immunotherapy in medical oncology. There is good preclinical and clinical data suggesting that immune-based approaches may be beneficial for the treatment of patients with HCC. One should not forget that HCC is an inflammation-induced cancer and therefore may be a good candidate for immune-based approaches. As a matter of fact, HBV vaccination can be considered the first successful preventive cancer vaccine. The increasing interest on immune-based approaches is reflected by an increased number of publications investigating immunological mechanisms in HCC (Fig. 1). Moreover, initial clinical trials testing immune checkpoint inhibitors have revealed positive results and led to the first phase III trial testing an immune checkpoint inhibitor in the first-line setting in HCC. In this book we would like to provide the reader with a solid immunological background making it easier to better understand the rational and basic mechanisms in liver cancer immunotherapy, summarize latest data from clinical trials testing immune-based approaches, and finally provide some insights about the future of immunotherapy in liver cancer.

Bethesda, May 17, 2017

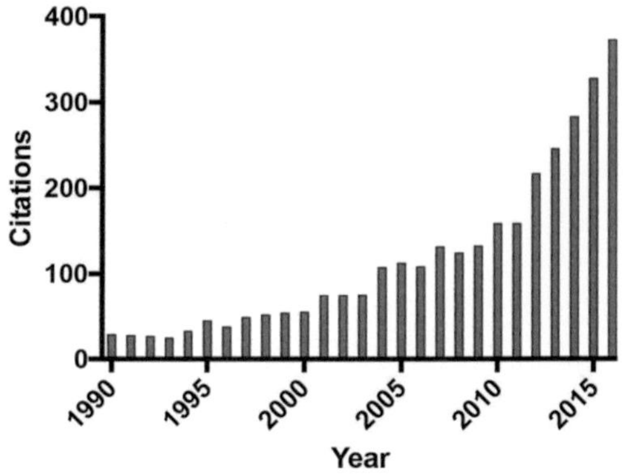

Fig. 1 Number of hits in PubMed per year as a result for "hepatocellular AND immune" search

Chapter 1
Vaccine Approaches in Hepatocellular Carcinoma

Maria Tagliamonte, Maria Lina Tornesello, Franco M. Buonaguro, and Luigi Buonaguro

Abbreviations

ABC	ATP-binding cassette
AFP	α-fetoprotein
APCs	antigen-presenting cells
APVAC	actively personalized vaccine
ASR	age-standardized rates
ATP	adenosine triphosphate
CIK	Cytokine-Induced NK-Like T Cells
CRC	colorectal cancer
CT	cancer testis
CTL	cytotoxic T lymphocytes
DAMPs	damage-associated molecular patterns
DCs	dendritic cells
GB	glioblastoma
GM-CSF	granulocyte-macrophage colony-stimulating factor
GPC-3	Glypican-3
HAIC	hepatic arterial infusion chemotherapy
HBV	hepatitis B virus
HCC	hepatocellular carcinoma
HCV	hepatitis C virus
hTERT	human telomerase reverse transcriptase
IFNγ	interferon gamma
IHC	immunohistochemistry
IL-10	interleukin 10

M. Tagliamonte • M.L. Tornesello • F.M. Buonaguro • L. Buonaguro (✉)
Laboratory of Molecular Biology and Viral Oncogenesis Unit, National Cancer Institute "Fond. G. Pascale", 80131 Naples, Italy
e-mail: l.buonaguro@istitutotumori.na.it

T.F. Greten (ed.), *Immunotherapy of Hepatocellular Carcinoma*,
DOI 10.1007/978-3-319-64958-0_1

LAK	limphokine-activated killer cells
LSECs	liver sinusoidal endothelial cells
MAGE-1*	Melanoma-associated antigen 1*
MDSCs	myeloid-derived suppressor cells
MHC I and II	Major Histocompatibility Class – I and II molecules
MRP3	Multidrug resistance-associated protein 3
OS	overall survival
PD-L1	Programmed death-ligand 1
PGE2	prostaglandin E2
RCC	renal cell cancer
RF	radiofrequency
SSX-2	synovial sarcoma X
TAAs	Tumor associated antigens
TACE	trans-arterial chemoembolization
TGF-β	transforming growth factor beta
Th	T helper cells
Tregs	T regulatory cells
TTP	time to progression
TTSP	time to symptomatic progression

1.1 Introduction

Hepatocellular carcinoma (HCC) is the most common liver malignancy, representing the third and the fifth leading cause of death from cancer worldwide in men and women, respectively.

The main risk factor for the development of HCC is the hepatitis B and C virus (HBV and HCV) infection; non-viral causes play a minor etiopathogenetic role. The main risk factor for the development of HCC is the hepatitis B and C virus (HBV and HCV) infection; non-viral causes play a minor etiopathogenetic role [1]. A range of therapies are used in the management of HCC according to the extent and severity of liver disease, but none of them shows a sufficient efficacy and the overall prognosis is poor with a 5-year survival rate of approximately 5–6% [2, 3]. The only effective strategy is represented by the preventive vaccine for the hepatitis B virus (HBV). Indeed, it prevents the establishment of a chronic infection by HBV and, consequently, the development of the HBV-related HCC [4]. In this regards, the preventive anti-HBV vaccine is considered the first preventive cancer vaccine introduced in the medicine practice.

Different immune-based therapeutic strategies targeting HCC have been evaluated in clinical trials with limited results, including immunomodulators (e.g. cytokines, ILs, chemokines) [5–7] and adoptive immunotherapy (e.g. LAK, CIK) [8, 9].

In this framework, a therapeutic cancer vaccine may represent an effective strategy to cure HCC. Unlike several other cancers, only few cancer vaccine trials for

HCC have been conducted so far with yet modest results [10–12], indicating that improvements in several aspects need to be implemented.

In particular, identification of novel specific tumor antigens, evaluation of delivery systems and combinatorial strategies to counteract the immunosuppressive microenvironment could result in unprecedented clinical outcomes with great beneficial effect for HCC patients.

1.1.1 Therapeutic Cancer Vaccines

Vaccines have been traditionally developed to prevent viral and bacterial diseases in healthy subjects (preventive vaccines). To this aim, they are based on foreign "non-self" antigens to induce a protective long-lasting immunological memory against a pathogen, which will swiftly respond to a subsequent infection by that specific pathogen and neutralize its effects in vivo. More recently, the concept of vaccine has been applied also to therapeutic strategies for patients affected by a disease including cancer (therapeutic cancer vaccines). In this case, they are based on internal "self" antigens specifically or preferentially expressed on tumor cells (tumor-associated antigens, TAAs) to elicit a therapeutic long-lasting immunological memory against the tumor cells. The immune response against the TAAs is more difficult to be elicited given that they are affected by central T-cell tolerance which avoids an auto- immunity against self own antigens. Preventive and therapeutic vaccines, in general, are sought to induce a distinct immune response: humoral antibody-mediated (preventive vaccines) and cytotoxic cellular-mediated (therapeutic vaccines).

Therapeutic cancer vaccine antigens are delivered in vivo according to different strategies (e.g. whole tumor lysates, full proteins, peptides, RNA, DNA), processed by antigen presenting cells (APCs) and presented to the effector T cells [13]. In particular, antigens are processed in short peptides (9–15 aa long) and coupled to the molecules of the Major Histocompatibility Class – I and II (MHC class I and II) to stimulate CD8+ T cytotoxic cells and CD4+ T helper, respectively. Cancer vaccine formulations always include immune stimulating molecules (i.e. adjuvants) which potentiate the effects of APCs in inducing the activation of effector T cells against the specific antigens coupled to the MHC molecules [14].

1.1.2 Target Antigens in Cancer Vaccines for HCC

Requirement for development of a cancer vaccine is the identification of specific tumor associated antigens (TAAs). In particular, cancer vaccines for HCC have been developed with either whole tumor lysates or individual antigens which, however, are not strictly specific to HCC. Few of such cancer vaccines have been evaluated in clinical trials which have provided disappointing results (Fig. 1.1).

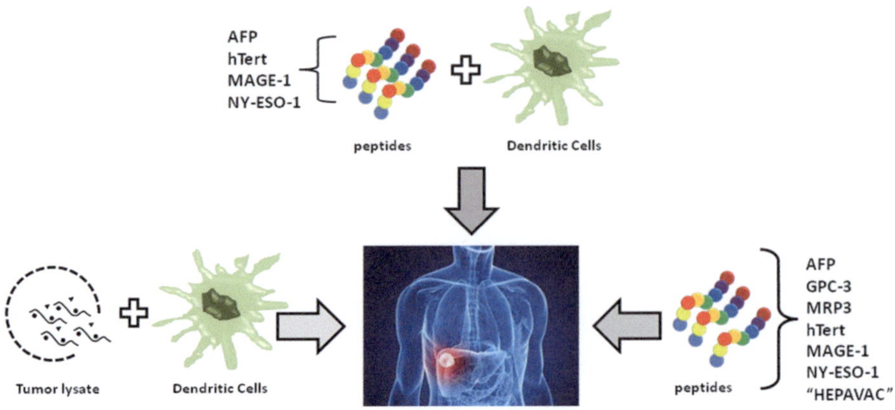

Fig. 1.1 HCC cancer vaccines tested in clinical trials. Schematic representation of the different cancer vaccine approaches and antigens evaluated in HCC patients in clinical trials

1.1.2.1 Whole Tumor Lysate

Tumor lysates have the advantage of including all potential tumor-associated antigens (TAAs) expressed by the tumor, together with adjuvanting molecules and damage-associated molecular patterns (DAMPs), to elicit a broad anti-tumor immune response. Tumor lysates are efficiently processed by professional antigen-presenting cells (APCs) (i.e. dendritic cells – DCs) and several tumor antigens are presented to $CD4^+$ T helper cells stimulating a strong polyclonal T cell response. This provides cognate help to $CD8^+$ T cells for generating a more robust anti-tumor immunity and long-term memory. Tumor lysates can be administered directly to patients to target DCs *in vivo* or pulsed onto DCs *ex vivo* and subsequently administrated to patients [15]. Such unbiased strategy eliminates the risk of selecting only specific TAAs which may not be the most relevant. The drawback of using tumor lysates is the "dilution and confounding factors" due to the low representation of such TAAs among the vast predominance of cellular self-antigens. This may result either in a poor effective elicitation of anti-tumor immune response or even in a competing immune suppressive effect (Table 1.1).

Early phase trials of DC vaccination have been conducted in the setting of advanced HCC using autologous DCs pulsed ex vivo with lysates derived from autologous liver cancer tumor cells or HepG2 cell line.

1.1.2.2 Autologous Tumor Lysate

A trial using DC loaded with autologous tumor lysate was conducted by Lee et al. [16]. Thirty-one patients with advanced HCC were enrolled in the study. DCs, derived from peripheral blood monocytes, were pulsed with autologous tumor lysates. The first 14 patients were treated with a pulsed regimen characterized by

Table 1.1 List of cancer vaccines evaluated in HCC patients

Antigen	Vaccine strategy	Clinical phase	Nr. patients	References
Autologous tumor lysate	DC pulsed	Phase I	31	Lee et al. [16]
Tumor cell line lysate	DC pulsed	Phase II	35	Palmer et al. [17]
	DC pulsed	Phase I	15	El Ansary et al. [18]
AFP	Peptides	Phase I	6	Butterfield et al. [27]
	Peptide DC pulsed	Phase I/II	10	Butterfield et al. [28]
	DNA + AdV	N/A	2	Butterfield et al. [29]
Glypican-3	Peptides	Phase I	33	Sawada et al. [33]
	Peptides	Phase II	41	Sawada et al. [34]
	MoAb	Phase I	20	Zhu et al. [35]
	MoAb	Phase II	125	Abou-Alfa et al. [36]
MRP-3	Peptide	Phase I	12	Mizukoshi et al. [39]
hTERT	Peptide	Phase II	40	Greten et al. [54, 100]
MAGE-1, AFP, NY-ESO-1	Peptide DC pulsed	Phase I	5	Tada et al. [48]
	Peptide DC pulsed	Phase I/Iia	12	Lee et al. [49]

DC dendritic cells, *AdV* adenovirus, *MoAb* Monoclonal antibody

five administration of DC vaccine intravenously at weekly intervals. The other 17 patients underwent monthly boost vaccinations after the initial 5-weeks pulsed therapy. Overall, the DC vaccination showed to be safe. Out of the 31 treated patients, 4 (12.9%) exhibited partial response and 17 (54.8%) had stable disease. Ten patients (32.3%) had progressive disease. Patients treated with pulsed and boosted therapy had much better 1-year survival rates than those treated by pulsed therapy alone (63.3 ± 12.0% vs. 10.7 ± 9.4%; $p < 0.001$). Overall, results were promising providing a ground for improvements.

1.1.2.3 HepG2 Cell Line Lysate

A phase II clinical trial investigating the safety and efficacy of vaccination with autologous DCs pulsed ex vivo with a liver tumor cell line lysate (HepG2) in patients with advanced HCC was reported by Palmer et al., [17]. Twenty-five patients received at least three doses of DC vaccinations each at 3-week intervals without signs of toxicity and were assessed clinically for response. An effect on disease, combining partial response and stable disease >3 months, was observed in 7 patients (28%). Only in 1 patient such effect was associated with a 90% reduction in serum α-fetoprotein (AFP). T cell responses specific to the vaccine or to AFP was induced by DC vaccination.

A further trial was conducted to evaluate safety and efficacy of a similar HepG2-pulsed DC vaccine [18]. Thirty patients with advanced HCC were randomized in two groups. Group 1 received a single administration of DC vaccination, Group 2 received supportive treatment. DC vaccination was safe. Partial response was observed in 2 patients (13.3%), stable disease in 9 patients (60%) and 4 patients (26.7%) showed progressive disease. The median survival time in Group 1 was 7 months compared to 4 months in Group 2.

Overall, DC vaccination loaded ex vivo with tumor lysate (autologous or cell line) shows safety and signs of efficacy which require improvements and further investigation on much large number of patients.

1.1.3 Individual Tumor Associated Antigen Vaccines

Cancer vaccines based on individual TAAs elicit a very specific anti-tumor effector and memory cell response. Indeed, such an approach eliminates the "dilution and confounding factors" characteristic of the whole tumor lysates by immunizing patients with large amounts of a desired TAA and eliciting a specific focused anti-tumor immune response.

Since the identification of the first human tumor antigen MAGE-1 [19], a large number of shared and unique TAAs have been and are constantly described [20, 21] (http://cancerimmunity.org/peptide/). Shared TAAs are currently classified as (i) cancer-testis (CT) antigens, (ii) differentiation antigens, and (iii) widely occurring, overexpressed antigens.

Cancer vaccines are mostly based on peptides covering a single cancer-testis or differentiation TAA, and most of them have been shown to induce a high frequency of specific T cells with limited clinical outcome [22, 23]. Several possible reasons may account for such unsatisfactory results, including immune tolerance induced by shared TAAs [24] and narrowed specificity of $CD8^+$ T cell response, resulting in limited immunological efficacy and induction of immune escape mechanisms [25, 26].

Concerning HCC, very few early phase clinical trials based on single TAA have been conducted in the setting of advanced HCC targeting antigens over-expressed in many HCC.

1.1.3.1 a-Fetoprotein (AFP)

Alpha fetoprotein (AFP) is an oncofetal antigen over-expressed in most HCCs offering an attractive target for HCC-specific immunotherapy approaches. The first pilot phase I clinical trial indicated that four specific AFP peptides are able to elicit a T cell response response in HCC patients, regardless the high circulating levels of AFP [27]. The mix of the four peptides was then used to pulse autologous DCs and evaluated in a phase I/II clinical trial in 10 AFP-positive HCC patients. At the end of the protocol, 6 of 10 subjects showed both expansion of AFP-specific T cells as well as increased IFNγ-producing AFP-specific Tcell responses to at least one of the peptides included in the mix [28].

In order to overcome the HLA restriction associated with a peptide-based approach, the full length AFP was tested in two HCC patients using a DNA prime – Adenovirus boost vaccine strategy. The vaccine was safe, well tolerated and both patients showed immunologic evidence of immunization. At the end of the protocol, the patients' AFP levels remained within the normal range and the level of AFP-specific CD8+ T cells remained high. Both patients showed immunologic evidence of immunization, but HCC recurred in 9 or 18 months [29]. Overall, cancer vaccines based on AFP have provided results in early clinical trials which do not support conduction of large efficacy randomized controlled trials.

1.1.3.2 Glypican-3 (GPC3)

Glypican-3 (GPC3) is a member of the glypican family of heparan sulfate proteoglycans, it is overexpressed in about 80% of HCC cases and is correlated with a poor prognosis [30–32]. Given such a specific expression pattern, GPC3 is considered a good target for HCC-specific immunotherapies. Two immunogenic HLA-A24 and HLA-A02 restricted GPC3 peptides have been identified and used for developing a therapeutic cancer vaccine for HCC. The safety of such a vaccine was evaluated in 33 patients with advanced HCC in a nonrandomized, open-label, phase I clinical trial. GPC3 vaccination was well-tolerated and 30 out 33 (91%) patients showed a GPC3-specific CTL response. One patient showed a partial response, and 19 patients showed stable disease 2 months after initiation of treatment. OS was significantly longer in patients with high GPC3-specific CTL frequencies than in those with low frequencies ($p = 0.033$) [33].

Based on such results, a phase II clinical study has been performed evaluating the GPC3 peptide vaccine in 41 HCC patients in an adjuvanting setting. Ten vaccinations were administered for 1 year after the standard treatment. The combination between surgery plus vaccination resulted in a lower recurrence rate compare to surgery alone (28.6% vs. 54.3% and 39.4% vs. 54.5% at 1 and 2 y, respectively; $p = 0.346, 0.983$). Moreover, the GPC3 expression on tumor strongly correlated with the recurrence rate at 1 year [34].

More recently a humanized monoclonal antibody against GPC3 (e.g. GC33, Codrituzumab) has been evaluated in a first-in-man Phase I clinical trial to assess its safety, tolerability, and pharmacokinetics in patients with advanced HCC [35]. A dose-escalating protocol was evaluated in 20 patients showing a safety profile. Stable disease was seen in 4 patients which exhibited a high intratumor GPC3 expression. Moreover, the median time to progression was significantly longer in patients with tumors expressing high levels of GPC3 than in patients with low GPC3 expression.

A randomized phase II trial with Codrituzumab was conducted in 185 advanced HCC patients who had failed prior systemic therapy. Patients were stratified based on GPC3 expression by IHC. Primary endpoint was progression free survival. Secondary endpoints included overall survival (OS), tolerability, pharmacokinetics, and an exploratory endpoint in biomarkers analysis. The results showed that

Codrituzumab failed in improving free survival and overall survival vs. the placebo group [36]. Such results do not support conduction of large efficacy randomized controlled trials.

1.1.3.3 Multidrug Resistance-Associated Protein 3 (MRP3)

Multidrug resistance-associated protein 3 (MRP3) is a carrier-type transport protein belonging to the ABC transporters. Its function is to transport substances against a concentration gradient in an ATP energy-dependent manner [37]. Among different tumor cells, MRP3 is highly expressed in HCC tissue and MRP3-specific cytotoxic T cells (CTLs) can be induced with cytotoxic activity against HCC cells overexpressing MRP3 [38]. Based on these observation, a phase I clinical trial has been recently conducted in HCC patients to evaluate safety and immunogenicity of a MRP3-derived peptide (MRP3765). Twelve hepatocellular carcinoma (HCC) patients treated with hepatic arterial infusion chemotherapy (HAIC) were enrolled and received three vaccine administrations weekly. The vaccination was well tolerated, no serious adverse reactions were observed and a MRP3-specific immunity was elicited in 8/12 patients. One patient showed a partial response, nine showed a stable disease, and two showed a progressive disease. The median overall survival time was 14.0 months [39]. These results indicate the feasibility of a MRP3-derived peptide vaccine and the potential efficacy should be further evaluated in additional studies.

1.1.3.4 Cancer-Testis Antigens

Cancer-testis (CT) antigens are tumor-associated antigens characterized by the expression limited to tumor tissue and testis [40]. Several CT have been identified in the last years and are considered an optimal target for cancer immunotherapy approaches [41]. Among such a family of TAAs, an increased mRNA expression of some of them has been detected in a variable percentage of HCC tissues. NY-ESO-1 has been detected in about 30% of HCCs [42] and a specific humoral and cellular response has been identified in about 12% of HCC patients [43]. Another study investigated the expression of 10 different CT genes in 21 HCC samples. Four samples did not express any of the CT genes tested, 17 (81%) expressed at least one, 9 (43%) coexpressed two, four (19%) coexpressed four, three (14%) coexpressed five and one coexpressed 8 of the 10 CT genes tested [44]. Spontaneous T cell response against specific CT has been detected in HCC patients, namely SSX-2 and MAGE-A10 [45] as well as melanoma antigen-encoding genes (MAGE A1- A6) [46].

More recently, the spontaneous $CD8^+$ T-cell responses specific for MAGE-1, together with AFP, GPC-3 and NY-ESO-1 has been assessed in a large cohort of HCC patients. The results showed that almost 50% of patients did not show any T cell response against any of the evaluated TAAs; 23% of patients reacted against only one of the TAAs; 11.5% against two TAAs; 10.5 against three TAAs and 6.3% against all 4 TAAs. Overall, 66.6% of HCC patients showed spontaneous $CD8^+$ T-cell responses against MAGE-1, AFP and GPC-3 [47]. The three TAAs have been used in a subsequent DC vaccine formulation which has been evaluated in early stage clinical trial in 5 HCC patients. The vaccine was safe and well-tolerated over 6 administrations, eliciting T cell responses against the three TAAs. However, clinical benefit was observed in one of the 5 patients [48]. More recently, the same DC vaccine formulation has been evaluated in a phase I/IIa study in 12 HCC patients who were tumor-free after primary treatments. Anti-tumor response was detected in all patients with a good correlation between cellular response and delayed tumour recurrence up to 24 weeks after DC vaccination. The median time of TTP was 36.6 months in the DC-vaccination group and 11.8 months in the control group [49].

1.1.3.5 Human Telomerase Reverse Transcriptase (hTERT)

Human telomerase reverse transcriptase (hTERT) is the catalytic enzyme required for telomere elongation and is expressed in a wide range of human cancers, including HCC [50–52]. The telomerase-derived peptide GV1001 has been identified as the best antigen for immunotherapy strategies targeting hTERT [53]. GV1001 in combination with GM-CSF was evaluated in a phase II clinical trial in 40 advanced HCC patients. Vaccination was preceded by a single administration with cyclophosphamide and was well tolerated. No GV1001 specific immune responses were detected after vaccination and none of the patients had a complete or partial response to treatment. 17 patients (45.9%) showed a stable disease 6 months after initiation of treatment. The median TTP was 57.0 days; the median TTSP was estimated to be 358.0 days [54].

Overall, trials have been conducted to examine the clinical response to vaccines based on individual TAAs but the clinical outcomes were not satisfactory and need further investigation to improve efficacy.

1.2 Overcoming Limiting Factors in Immunotherapy Approaches for HCC

The disappointing clinical responses observed in the different early clinical trials described above can be ascribed to two main reasons. One is the target TAAs used in such vaccines which are not specific to HCC and are not expressed in the totality of liver cancer cells. Moreover, they have been used a single target which may easily lead to an immunological escape. The second one is the strong intrinsic immune suppressive microenvironment characterizing the liver which may represent a major impediment to an effective anti-tumor activity elicited by a therapeutic cancer vaccine [10].

1.2.1 HCC-Specific Tumor Associated Antigens (TAAs)

Identification of HCC-specific TAAs and/or epitopes need to be identified, both HLA class I and II restricted, in order to induce both $CD4^+$ T helper and $CD8^+$ T cytotoxic responses [55–58]. Novel TAAs can be identified according to three different experimental approaches.

The cellular approach is based on elution of antigenic peptides from target cells, determination of peptide sequences by reverse phase HPLC fractionation and Edman degradation, identification of peptides by sensitive mass spectroscopy (reviewed in [59, 60]). The genetic approach is based on expression cloning of libraries derived from tumor cells. (reviewed in [61]).

The third approach is based on *in silico* prediction methods, which is named "reverse immunology" [62]. Potential HLA-associated peptides are predicted from full-length protein sequences by immune-informatics algorithms [63–70]. However, such algorithms cannot take into account the complexity of the whole biological process leading to generation of peptides by the proteasome, their coupling to HLA molecules and presentation on the cellular surface. To this aim, integration of multiple high-throughput "omics" technologies is needed (reviewed in [71, 72]). Rammensee and colleagues proposed a strategy based on a combination of the described approaches defined as "Tuebingen approach" [73]. The combination of genomics, HLA peptide repertoire analysis by liquid chromatography-coupled mass spectrometry ("peptidomics") and classical as well as novel T-cell assays has allowed the identification of HLA ligands from frozen primary tumor material, selection of the tumor associated peptides and their immunological validation [74]. Such an integrated strategy has been employed to identify the HLA ligandome for glioblastoma (GB) [75], renal cell cancer (RCC) and colorectal cancer (CRC). Cancer vaccines based on peptides identified with this strategy have been developed and phase I-III clinical trials have been conducted in patients affected by GB, RCC and CRC [76–78].

The same strategy is currently pursued for identification of shared "off-the-shelf" HCC-specific antigens within the HEPAVAC project (www.hepavac.eu) [11]. Novel HCC-associated antigens have been identified and a multi-epitope, multi-HLA peptide vaccine has been produced. The vaccine, indeed, is a cocktail including 13 HLA class I (A*02 and A*24) and 5 HLA class II peptides, to raise a $CD4^+$ T helper and $CD8^+$ CTL response as well as to avoid a possible immunological escape. A phase I/II clinical trial is going to start in Q1 2017 to assess safety and immunogenicity in early-intermediate stage HCC patients undergoing surgical and/or loco-regional treatments. The vaccination protocol will an actively personalized vaccine (APVAC) in a subset of vaccinees. Patient-specific HCC-specific neo-antigens will be selected according to integration of genomics, transcriptomics and HLA ligandomics analyses. Both the "off-the-shelf" and the personalized vaccine will be combined with a novel and potent RNA-based immunomodulator (RNAdjuvant®) which is based on a noncoding, long-chain RNA molecule able to induce balanced, long-lasting immune responses resulting in a strong anti-tumor activity [79–81].

1.2.2 Liver Immunosuppressive Environment

The intrinsinc tolerogenicity of liver is the due to resident subsets of phagocytic cells which have been identified to play a role as "tolerogenic" antigen presenting cells (APCs): liver sinusoidal endothelial cells (LSECs); Kupffer cells and liver dendritic cells (DCs). LSECs inhibit T cell response [82, 83] and induce CD4+ T cell tolerance and death [84]. Kupffer cells produce the anti-inflammatory molecules transforming growth factor beta (TGF-β), IL-10, prostaglandin E2 (PGE2), as well as express the inhibitory molecule PD-L1 [85–87]. Liver-resident DCs show an IL-10-secreting phenotype [88–90], inducing Th2 polarization of CD4+ T cells [91], regulatory T cell (Treg) induction and poor antigen recall responses [92, 93].

Such inherent immunological uniqueness needs to be taken into high account to significantly improve the immune response elicited by active cancer immunotherapies. Combinatorial protocols combining specific immunotherapy approaches with immune stimulatory strategies counterbalancing the immune-suppressive tumor environment would be of high efficacy (reviewed in [94]). To this aim, several lines of evidence suggest that combination of immunotherapy and cancer standard-of-care therapies (i.e. chemotherapy) may provide better results than individual treatments (reviewed in [95, 96]).

Cytotoxic chemotherapy has been recently shown to generate a favorable immune environment and potentiate effects of anticancer vaccines (reviewed in [97]). Indeed, cyclophosphamide is toxic to immunosuppressive Treg cells and a metronomic regimen has been shown to improve cancer vaccine efficacy [98–102]. Similarly, gemcitabine selectively kills myeloid-derived suppressor cells (MDSCs) *in vitro* and *in vivo* [103], and has been shown to improve immune response to cancer vaccines [104–106]. Docetaxel has been reported to modulate different cell subsets, enhancing CD8+ function and deleting Tregs [107] and has been evaluated in several human clinical trials showing enhancement of immune response to cancer vaccine [108, 109].

Specifically concerning the HCC, a single clinical trial has evaluated a combination of low dose cyclophosphamide with a telomerase peptide (GV1001) vaccination with limited results [54]. Such a specific combinatorial strategy needs to be evaluated in much more details in HCC. However, considering all the data generated for other cancer models, it is reasonable to predict that chemotherapeutic agents may improve the efficacy of cancer vaccines also in this tumor setting.

1.3 Concluding Remarks

HCC has a poor prognosis for the lack of an effective therapy. Development of a cancer vaccine as therapeutic strategy is of high relevance. However, until now the efficacy of cancer vaccines evaluated in advanced HCC patients in early phase clinical trials has been disappointing. Two are the main aspects which needs to be addressed in more details for improving clinical outcomes with great beneficial effect for HCC patients. The first is increasing the knowledge on molecular and antigenic characteristics of HCC, to identify more specific and immunogenic tumor-associated antigens. The second is testing the potential benefits of the combinatorial strategies, to counterbalance the immune-suppressive environment and increase the vaccine immunogenicity. The EU-funded HEPVAC project is currently addressing such aspects and the clinical trial about to start with the multi-epitope, multi-HLA peptide vaccine will hopefully provide relevant results for the HCC patients.

Conflict of Interests The authors declare that they have no competing interests.

References

1. Forner A, Llovet JM, Bruix J. Hepatocellular carcinoma. Lancet. 2012;379(9822):1245–55.
2. European Association for the Study of the Liver EOfRaToC. EASL-EORTC clinical practice guidelines: management of hepatocellular carcinoma. J Hepatol. 2012;56(4):908–43.
3. Fong ZV, Tanabe KK. The clinical management of hepatocellular carcinoma in the United States, Europe, and Asia: a comprehensive and evidence-based comparison and review. Cancer. 2014;120(18):2824–38.
4. Qu C, Chen T, Fan C, Zhan Q, Wang Y, Lu J, et al. Efficacy of neonatal HBV vaccination on liver cancer and other liver diseases over 30-year follow-up of the Qidong hepatitis B intervention study: a cluster randomized controlled trial. PLoS Med. 2014;11(12):e1001774.
5. Chen LT, Chen MF, Li LA, Lee PH, Jeng LB, Lin DY, et al. Long-term results of a randomized, observation-controlled, phase III trial of adjuvant interferon Alfa-2b in hepatocellular carcinoma after curative resection. Ann Surg. 2012;255(1):8–17.
6. Llovet JM, Sala M, Castells L, Suarez Y, Vilana R, Bianchi L, et al. Randomized controlled trial of interferon treatment for advanced hepatocellular carcinoma. Hepatology. 2000;31(1):54–8.
7. Sangro B, Mazzolini G, Ruiz J, Herraiz M, Quiroga J, Herrero I, et al. Phase I trial of intratumoral injection of an adenovirus encoding interleukin-12 for advanced digestive tumors. J Clin Oncol. 2004;22(8):1389–97.
8. Haruta I, Yamauchi K, Aruga A, Komatsu T, Takasaki K, Hayashi N, et al. Analytical study of the clinical response to two distinct adoptive immunotherapies for advanced hepatocellular carcinoma: comparison between LAK cell and CTL therapy. J Immunother Emphasis Tumor Immunol. 1996;19(3):218–23.
9. Li X, Dai D, Song X, Liu J, Zhu L, Xu W. A meta-analysis of cytokine-induced killer cells therapy in combination with minimally invasive treatment for hepatocellular carcinoma. Clin Res Hepatol Gastroenterol. 2014;38(5):583–91.
10. Buonaguro L, Petrizzo A, Tagliamonte M, Tornesello ML, Buonaguro FM. Challenges in cancer vaccine development for hepatocellular carcinoma. J Hepatol. 2013;59(4):897–903.
11. Buonaguro L, HEPAVAC Consortium. Developments in cancer vaccines for hepatocellular carcinoma. Cancer Immunol Immunother. 2016;65(1):93–9.
12. Sun Z, Zhu Y, Xia J, Sawakami T, Kokudo N, Zhang N. Status of and prospects for cancer vaccines against hepatocellular carcinoma in clinical trials. Biosci Trends. 2016;10(2):85–91.
13. Melief CJ, Van HT, Arens R, Ossendorp F, van der Burg SH. Therapeutic cancer vaccines. J Clin Invest. 2015;125(9):3401–12.
14. Di Pasquale A, Preiss S, Tavares Da SF, Garcon N. Vaccine adjuvants: from 1920 to 2015 and beyond. Vaccines (Basel). 2015;3(2):320–43.

15. Chiang CL, Coukos G, Kandalaft LE. Whole tumor antigen vaccines: where are we? Vaccines (Basel). 2015;3(2):344–72.
16. Lee WC, Wang HC, Hung CF, Huang PF, Lia CR, Chen MF. Vaccination of advanced hepatocellular carcinoma patients with tumor lysate-pulsed dendritic cells: a clinical trial. J Immunother. 2005;28(5):496–504.
17. Palmer DH, Midgley RS, Mirza N, Torr EE, Ahmed F, Steele JC, et al. A phase II study of adoptive immunotherapy using dendritic cells pulsed with tumor lysate in patients with hepatocellular carcinoma. Hepatology. 2009;49(1):124–32.
18. El Ansary M, Mogawer S, Elhamid SA, Alwakil S, Aboelkasem F, Sabaawy HE, et al. Immunotherapy by autologous dendritic cell vaccine in patients with advanced HCC. J Cancer Res Clin Oncol. 2013;139(1):39–48.
19. van der Bruggen P, Traversari C, Chomez P, Lurquin C, De PE, Van den EB, et al. A gene encoding an antigen recognized by cytolytic T lymphocytes on a human melanoma. Science. 1991;254(5038):1643–7.
20. Buonaguro L, Petrizzo A, Tornesello ML, Buonaguro FM. Translating tumor antigens into cancer vaccines. Clin Vaccine Immunol. 2011;18(1):23–34.
21. Tagliamonte M, Petrizzo A, Tornesello ML, Buonaguro FM, Buonaguro L. Antigen-specific vaccines for cancer treatment. Hum Vaccin Immunother. 2014;10(11):3332–46.
22. Xiao YF, Jie MM, Li BS, Hu CJ, Xie R, Tang B, et al. Peptide-Based Treatment: A Promising Cancer Therapy. J Immunol Res. 2015;2015:761820.
23. Parmiani G, Russo V, Maccalli C, Parolini D, Rizzo N, Maio M. Peptide-based vaccines for cancer therapy. Hum Vaccin Immunother. 2014;18:10(11).
24. Slingluff CL Jr, Chianese-Bullock KA, Bullock TN, Grosh WW, Mullins DW, Nichols L, et al. Immunity to melanoma antigens: from self-tolerance to immunotherapy. Adv Immunol. 2006;90:243–95.
25. Rivoltini L, Canese P, Huber V, Iero M, Pilla L, Valenti R, et al. Escape strategies and reasons for failure in the interaction between tumour cells and the immune system: how can we tilt the balance towards immune-mediated cancer control? Expert Opin Biol Ther. 2005;5(4):463–76.
26. Peggs KS, Quezada SA, Allison JP. Cell intrinsic mechanisms of T-cell inhibition and application to cancer therapy. Immunol Rev. 2008;224:141–65.
27. Butterfield LH, Ribas A, Meng WS, Dissette VB, Amarnani S, Vu HT, et al. T-cell responses to HLA-A*0201 immunodominant peptides derived from alpha-fetoprotein in patients with hepatocellular cancer. Clin Cancer Res. 2003;9(16 Pt 1):5902–8.
28. Butterfield LH, Ribas A, Dissette VB, Lee Y, Yang JQ, De la RP, et al. A phase I/II trial testing immunization of hepatocellular carcinoma patients with dendritic cells pulsed with four alpha-fetoprotein peptides. Clin Cancer Res. 2006;12(9):2817–25.
29. Butterfield LH, Economou JS, Gamblin TC, Geller DA. Alpha fetoprotein DNA prime and adenovirus boost immunization of two hepatocellular cancer patients. J Transl Med. 2014;12:86.
30. Nakatsura T, Yoshitake Y, Senju S, Monji M, Komori H, Motomura Y, et al. Glypican-3, overexpressed specifically in human hepatocellular carcinoma, is a novel tumor marker. Biochem Biophys Res Commun. 2003;306(1):16–25.
31. Shirakawa H, Kuronuma T, Nishimura Y, Hasebe T, Nakano M, Gotohda N, et al. Glypican-3 is a useful diagnostic marker for a component of hepatocellular carcinoma in human liver cancer. Int J Oncol. 2009;34(3):649–56.
32. Shirakawa H, Suzuki H, Shimomura M, Kojima M, Gotohda N, Takahashi S, et al. Glypican-3 expression is correlated with poor prognosis in hepatocellular carcinoma. Cancer Sci. 2009;100(8):1403–7.
33. Sawada Y, Yoshikawa T, Nobuoka D, Shirakawa H, Kuronuma T, Motomura Y, et al. Phase I trial of a glypican-3-derived peptide vaccine for advanced hepatocellular carcinoma: immunologic evidence and potential for improving overall survival. Clin Cancer Res. 2012;18(13):3686–96.

34. Sawada Y, Yoshikawa T, Ofuji K, Yoshimura M, Tsuchiya N, Takahashi M, et al. Phase II study of the adjuvant therapy for hepatocellular carcinoma an adjuvant therapy for hepatocellular carcinoma patients. Oncoimmunology. 2016;5(5):e1129483.
35. Zhu AX, Gold PJ, El-Khoueiry AB, Abrams TA, Morikawa H, Ohishi N, et al. First-in-man phase I study of GC33, a novel recombinant humanized antibody against glypican-3, in patients with advanced hepatocellular carcinoma. Clin Cancer Res. 2013;19(4):920–8.
36. Abou-Alfa GK, Puig O, Daniele B, Kudo M, Merle P, Park JW, et al. Randomized phase II placebo controlled study of codrituzumab in previously treated patients with advanced hepatocellular carcinoma. J Hepatol. 2016;65(2):289–95.
37. Borst P, Elferink RO. Mammalian ABC transporters in health and disease. Annu Rev Biochem. 2002;71:537–92.
38. Mizukoshi E, Honda M, Arai K, Yamashita T, Nakamoto Y, Kaneko S. Expression of multidrug resistance-associated protein 3 and cytotoxic T cell responses in patients with hepatocellular carcinoma. J Hepatol. 2008;49(6):946–54.
39. Mizukoshi E, Nakagawa H, Kitahara M, Yamashita T, Arai K, Sunagozaka H, et al. Phase I trial of multidrug resistance-associated protein 3-derived peptide in patients with hepatocellular carcinoma. Cancer Lett. 2015;369(1):242–9.
40. Scanlan MJ, Gure AO, Jungbluth AA, Old LJ, Chen YT. Cancer/testis antigens: an expanding family of targets for cancer immunotherapy. Immunol Rev. 2002;188:22–32.
41. Gjerstorff MF, Andersen MH, Ditzel HJ. Oncogenic cancer/testis antigens: prime candidates for immunotherapy. Oncotarget. 2015;6(18):15772–87.
42. Chen CH, Chen GJ, Lee HS, Huang GT, Yang PM, Tsai LJ, et al. Expressions of cancer-testis antigens in human hepatocellular carcinomas. Cancer Lett. 2001;164(2):189–95.
43. Korangy F, Ormandy LA, Bleck JS, Klempnauer J, Wilkens L, Manns MP, et al. Spontaneous tumor-specific humoral and cellular immune responses to NY-ESO-1 in hepatocellular carcinoma. Clin Cancer Res. 2004;10(13):4332–41.
44. Luo G, Huang S, Xie X, Stockert E, Chen YT, Kubuschok B, et al. Expression of cancer-testis genes in human hepatocellular carcinomas. Cancer Immun. 2002;2:11.
45. Bricard G, Bouzourene H, Martinet O, Rimoldi D, Halkic N, Gillet M, et al. Naturally acquired MAGE-A10- and SSX-2-specific CD8+ T cell responses in patients with hepatocellular carcinoma. J Immunol. 2005;174(3):1709–16.
46. Zerbini A, Pilli M, Soliani P, Ziegler S, Pelosi G, Orlandini A, et al. Ex vivo characterization of tumor-derived melanoma antigen encoding gene-specific CD8+cells in patients with hepatocellular carcinoma. J Hepatol. 2004;40(1):102–9.
47. Flecken T, Schmidt N, Hild S, Gostick E, Drognitz O, Zeiser R, et al. Immunodominance and functional alterations of tumor-associated antigen-specific CD8+ T-cell responses in hepatocellular carcinoma. Hepatology. 2014;59(4):1415–26.
48. Tada F, Abe M, Hirooka M, Ikeda Y, Hiasa Y, Lee Y, et al. Phase I/II study of immunotherapy using tumor antigen-pulsed dendritic cells in patients with hepatocellular carcinoma. Int J Oncol. 2012;41(5):1601–9.
49. Lee JH, Lee Y, Lee M, Heo MK, Song JS, Kim KH, et al. A phase I/IIa study of adjuvant immunotherapy with tumour antigen-pulsed dendritic cells in patients with hepatocellular carcinoma. Br J Cancer. 2015;113(12):1666–76.
50. Meyerson M, Counter CM, Eaton EN, Ellisen LW, Steiner P, Caddle SD, et al. hEST2, the putative human telomerase catalytic subunit gene, is up-regulated in tumor cells and during immortalization. Cell. 1997;90(4):785–95.
51. Vonderheide RH, Hahn WC, Schultze JL, Nadler LM. The telomerase catalytic subunit is a widely expressed tumor-associated antigen recognized by cytotoxic T lymphocytes. Immunity. 1999;10(6):673–9.
52. Mizukoshi E, Nakamoto Y, Marukawa Y, Arai K, Yamashita T, Tsuji H, et al. Cytotoxic T cell responses to human telomerase reverse transcriptase in patients with hepatocellular carcinoma. Hepatology. 2006;43(6):1284–94.

53. Brunsvig PF, Aamdal S, Gjertsen MK, Kvalheim G, Markowski-Grimsrud CJ, Sve I, et al. Telomerase peptide vaccination: a phase I/II study in patients with non-small cell lung cancer. Cancer Immunol Immunother. 2006;55(12):1553–64.
54. Greten TF, Forner A, Korangy F, N'Kontchou G, Barget N, Ayuso C, et al. A phase II open label trial evaluating safety and efficacy of a telomerase peptide vaccination in patients with advanced hepatocellular carcinoma. BMC Cancer. 2010;10:209.
55. Hamilton SE, Wolkers MC, Schoenberger SP, Jameson SC. The generation of protective memory-like CD8+ T cells during homeostatic proliferation requires CD4+ T cells. Nat Immunol. 2006;7(5):475–81.
56. Hung K, Hayashi R, Lafond-Walker A, Lowenstein C, Pardoll D, Levitsky H. The central role of CD4(+) T cells in the antitumor immune response. J Exp Med. 1998;188(12):2357–68.
57. Janssen EM, Lemmens EE, Wolfe T, Christen U, von Herrath MG, Schoenberger SP. CD4+ T cells are required for secondary expansion and memory in CD8+ T lymphocytes. Nature. 2003;421(6925):852–6.
58. Pardoll DM, Topalian SL. The role of CD4+ T cell responses in antitumor immunity. Curr Opin Immunol. 1998;10(5):588–94.
59. Krishna S, Anderson KS. T-cell epitope discovery for therapeutic cancer vaccines. Methods Mol Biol. 2016;1403:779–96.
60. Comber JD, Philip R. MHC class I antigen presentation and implications for developing a new generation of therapeutic vaccines. Ther Adv Vaccines. 2014;2(3):77–89.
61. Coulie PG, Van den Eynde BJ, van der Bruggen P, Boon T. Tumour antigens recognized by T lymphocytes: at the core of cancer immunotherapy. Nat Rev Cancer. 2014;14(2):135–46.
62. Celis E, Tsai V, Crimi C, DeMars R, Wentworth PA, Chesnut RW, et al. Induction of anti-tumor cytotoxic T lymphocytes in normal humans using primary cultures and synthetic peptide epitopes. Proc Natl Acad Sci U S A. 1994;91(6):2105–9.
63. Rammensee H, Bachmann J, Emmerich NP, Bachor OA, Stevanovic S. SYFPEITHI: database for MHC ligands and peptide motifs. Immunogenetics. 1999;50(3–4):213–9.
64. Singh H, Raghava GP. ProPred: prediction of HLA-DR binding sites. Bioinformatics. 2001;17(12):1236–7.
65. Reche PA, Glutting JP, Reinherz EL. Prediction of MHC class I binding peptides using profile motifs. Hum Immunol. 2002;63(9):701–9.
66. Guan P, Hattotuwagama CK, Doytchinova IA, Flower DR. MHCPred 2.0: an updated quantitative T-cell epitope prediction server. Appl Bioinforma. 2006;5(1):55–61.
67. Bachinsky MM, Guillen DE, Patel SR, Singleton J, Chen C, Soltis DA, et al. Mapping and binding analysis of peptides derived from the tumor-associated antigen survivin for eight HLA alleles. Cancer Immun. 2005;5:6.
68. Carrasco PS, Zimic M, Nielsen M. Improved pan-specific MHC class I peptide-binding predictions using a novel representation of the MHC-binding cleft environment. Tissue Antigens. 2014;83(2):94–100.
69. Lundegaard C, Lund O, Buus S, Nielsen M. Major histocompatibility complex class I binding predictions as a tool in epitope discovery. Immunology. 2010 Jul;130(3):309–18.
70. Jorgensen KW, Rasmussen M, Buus S, Nielsen M. NetMHCstab – predicting stability of peptide-MHC-I complexes; impacts for cytotoxic T lymphocyte epitope discovery. Immunology. 2014;141(1):18–26.
71. O'Meara MM, Disis ML. Therapeutic cancer vaccines and translating vaccinomics science to the global health clinic: emerging applications toward proof of concept. OMICS. 2011;15(9):579–88.
72. Petrizzo A, Tagliamonte M, Tornesello M, Buonaguro FM, Buonaguro L. Systems vaccinology for cancer vaccine development. Expert Rev Vaccines. 2014;13(6):711–9.
73. Singh-Jasuja H, Emmerich NP, Rammensee HG. The Tubingen approach: identification, selection, and validation of tumor-associated HLA peptides for cancer therapy. Cancer Immunol Immunother. 2004;53(3):187–95.

74. Rammensee HG, Singh-Jasuja H. HLA ligandome tumor antigen discovery for personalized vaccine approach. Expert Rev Vaccines. 2013;12(10):1211–7.
75. Dutoit V, Herold-Mende C, Hilf N, Schoor O, Beckhove P, Bucher J, et al. Exploiting the glioblastoma peptidome to discover novel tumour-associated antigens for immunotherapy. Brain. 2012;135(Pt 4):1042–54.
76. Kuttruff S, Weinschenk T, Schoor O, Lindner J, Kutscher S, Maurer D, et al. Immune responses and association with clinical outcome of advanced colorectal cancer patients with the multi-peptide vaccine IMA910. J Clin Oncol 2012 ASCO Annual Meeting Proceedings 2012;30 suppl; abstr 2522.
77. Walter S, Weinschenk T, Stenzl A, Zdrojowy R, Pluzanska A, Szczylik C, et al. Multipeptide immune response to cancer vaccine IMA901 after single-dose cyclophosphamide associates with longer patient survival. Nat Med. 2012;18(8):1254–61.
78. Rini BI, Stenzl A, Zdrojowy R, Kogan M, Shkolnik M, Oudard S, et al. IMA901, a multipeptide cancer vaccine, plus sunitinib versus sunitinib alone, as first-line therapy for advanced or metastatic renal cell carcinoma (IMPRINT): a multicentre, open-label, randomised, controlled, phase 3 trial. Lancet Oncol. 2016;17(11):1599–611.
79. Heidenreich R, Fotin-Mleczek M, Baumhof P, Scheel B, Voss S, Kramps T, Kallen KJ. RNAdjuvant® is a novel potent adjuvant with a strong anti-tumor activity and a very favourable safety profile. Immunotherapy. 2012;35(9). Ref Type: Abstract.
80. Heidenreich R, Jasny E, Kowalczyk A, Lutz J, Probst J, Baumhof P, et al. A novel RNA-based adjuvant combines strong immunostimulatory capacities with a favorable safety profile. Int J Cancer. 2015;137:372–84.
81. Circelli L, Petrizzo A, Tagliamonte M, Heidenreich R, Tornesello ML, Buonaguro FM, et al. Immunological effects of a novel RNA-based adjuvant in liver cancer patients. Cancer Immunol Immunother. 2017;66(1):103–12.
82. Diehl L, Schurich A, Grochtmann R, Hegenbarth S, Chen L, Knolle PA. Tolerogenic maturation of liver sinusoidal endothelial cells promotes B7-homolog 1-dependent CD8+ T cell tolerance. Hepatology. 2008;47(1):296–305.
83. Tang L, Yang J, Liu W, Tang X, Chen J, Zhao D, et al. Liver sinusoidal endothelial cell lectin, LSECtin, negatively regulates hepatic T-cell immune response. Gastroenterology. 2009;137(4):1498–508.
84. Tokita D, Shishida M, Ohdan H, Onoe T, Hara H, Tanaka Y, et al. Liver sinusoidal endothelial cells that endocytose allogeneic cells suppress T cells with indirect allospecificity. J Immunol. 2006;177(6):3615–24.
85. Kuniyasu Y, Marfani SM, Inayat IB, Sheikh SZ, Mehal WZ. Kupffer cells required for high affinity peptide-induced deletion, not retention, of activated CD8+ T cells by mouse liver. Hepatology. 2004;39(4):1017–27.
86. You Q, Cheng L, Kedl RM, Ju C. Mechanism of T cell tolerance induction by murine hepatic Kupffer cells. Hepatology. 2008;48(3):978–90.
87. Wu K, Kryczek I, Chen L, Zou W, Welling TH. Kupffer cell suppression of CD8+ T cells in human hepatocellular carcinoma is mediated by B7-H1/programmed death-1 interactions. Cancer Res. 2009;69(20):8067–75.
88. Li G, Kim YJ, Broxmeyer HE. Macrophage colony-stimulating factor drives cord blood monocyte differentiation into IL-10(high)IL-12absent dendritic cells with tolerogenic potential. J Immunol. 2005;174(8):4706–17.
89. Rutella S, Danese S, Leone G. Tolerogenic dendritic cells: cytokine modulation comes of age. Blood. 2006;108(5):1435–40.
90. Bamboat ZM, Stableford JA, Plitas G, Burt BM, Nguyen HM, Welles AP, et al. Human liver dendritic cells promote T cell hyporesponsiveness. J Immunol. 2009;182(4):1901–11.
91. Khanna A, Morelli AE, Zhong C, Takayama T, Lu L, Thomson AW. Effects of liver-derived dendritic cell progenitors on Th1- and Th2-like cytokine responses in vitro and in vivo. J Immunol. 2000;164(3):1346–54.

92. Goubier A, Dubois B, Gheit H, Joubert G, Villard-Truc F, Asselin-Paturel C, et al. Plasmacytoid dendritic cells mediate oral tolerance. Immunity. 2008;29(3):464–75.
93. Dubois B, Joubert G, Gomez de AM, Gouanvic M, Goubier A, Kaiserlian D. Sequential role of plasmacytoid dendritic cells and regulatory T cells in oral tolerance. Gastroenterology. 2009;137(3):1019–28.
94. Tagliamonte M, Petrizzo A, Tornesello ML, Ciliberto G, Buonaguro FM, Buonaguro L. Combinatorial immunotherapy strategies for hepatocellular carcinoma. Curr Opin Immunol. 2016;39:103–13.
95. Hodge JW, Ardiani A, Farsaci B, Kwilas AR, Gameiro SR. The tipping point for combination therapy: cancer vaccines with radiation, chemotherapy, or targeted small molecule inhibitors. Semin Oncol. 2012;39(3):323–39.
96. Vanneman M, Dranoff G. Combining immunotherapy and targeted therapies in cancer treatment. Nat Rev Cancer. 2012;12(4):237–51.
97. Galluzzi L, Buque A, Kepp O, Zitvogel L, Kroemer G. Immunological effects of conventional chemotherapy and targeted anticancer agents. Cancer Cell. 2015;28(6):690–714.
98. Machiels JP, Reilly RT, Emens LA, Ercolini AM, Lei RY, Weintraub D, et al. Cyclophosphamide, doxorubicin, and paclitaxel enhance the antitumor immune response of granulocyte/macrophage-colony stimulating factor-secreting whole-cell vaccines in HER-2/neu tolerized mice. Cancer Res. 2001;61(9):3689–97.
99. Emens LA, Asquith JM, Leatherman JM, Kobrin BJ, Petrik S, Laiko M, et al. Timed sequential treatment with cyclophosphamide, doxorubicin, and an allogeneic granulocyte-macrophage colony-stimulating factor-secreting breast tumor vaccine: a chemotherapy dose-ranging factorial study of safety and immune activation. J Clin Oncol. 2009;27(35):5911–8.
100. Greten TF, Ormandy LA, Fikuart A, Hochst B, Henschen S, Horning M, et al. Low-dose cyclophosphamide treatment impairs regulatory T cells and unmasks AFP-specific CD4+ T-cell responses in patients with advanced HCC. J Immunother. 2010;33(2):211–8.
101. Hoon DS, Foshag LJ, Nizze AS, Bohman R, Morton DL. Suppressor cell activity in a randomized trial of patients receiving active specific immunotherapy with melanoma cell vaccine and low dosages of cyclophosphamide. Cancer Res. 1990;50(17):5358–64.
102. Slingluff CL Jr, Petroni GR, Chianese-Bullock KA, Smolkin ME, Ross MI, Haas NB, et al. Randomized multicenter trial of the effects of melanoma-associated helper peptides and cyclophosphamide on the immunogenicity of a multipeptide melanoma vaccine. J Clin Oncol. 2011;29(21):2924–32.
103. Suzuki E, Kapoor V, Jassar AS, Kaiser LR, Albelda SM. Gemcitabine selectively eliminates splenic Gr-1+/CD11b+ myeloid suppressor cells in tumor-bearing animals and enhances antitumor immune activity. Clin Cancer Res. 2005;11(18):6713–21.
104. Kaida M, Morita-Hoshi Y, Soeda A, Wakeda T, Yamaki Y, Kojima Y, et al. Phase 1 trial of Wilms tumor 1 (WT1) peptide vaccine and gemcitabine combination therapy in patients with advanced pancreatic or biliary tract cancer. J Immunother. 2011;34(1):92–9.
105. Yanagimoto H, Shiomi H, Satoi S, Mine T, Toyokawa H, Yamamoto T, et al. A phase II study of personalized peptide vaccination combined with gemcitabine for non-resectable pancreatic cancer patients. Oncol Rep. 2010;24(3):795–801.
106. Kimura Y, Tsukada J, Tomoda T, Takahashi H, Imai K, Shimamura K, et al. Clinical and immunologic evaluation of dendritic cell-based immunotherapy in combination with gemcitabine and/or S-1 in patients with advanced pancreatic carcinoma. Pancreas. 2012;41(2):195–205.
107. Garnett CT, Schlom J, Hodge JW. Combination of docetaxel and recombinant vaccine enhances T-cell responses and antitumor activity: effects of docetaxel on immune enhancement. Clin Cancer Res. 2008;14(11):3536–44.
108. Arlen PM, Pazdur M, Skarupa L, Rauckhorst M, Gulley JL. A randomized phase II study of docetaxel alone or in combination with PANVAC-V (vaccinia) and PANVAC-F (fowlpox) in patients with metastatic breast cancer (NCI 05-C-0229). Clin Breast Cancer. 2006;7(2):176–9.
109. Arlen PM, Gulley JL, Parker C, Skarupa L, Pazdur M, Panicali D, et al. A randomized phase II study of concurrent docetaxel plus vaccine versus vaccine alone in metastatic androgen-independent prostate cancer. Clin Cancer Res. 2006;12(4):1260–9.

Chapter 2
Natural Killer Cells in Hepatocellular Carcinoma: Anti-Tumor Effect and Therapeutic Potential

Elisabetta Cariani and Gabriele Missale

2.1 NK-Cell Function

As the principal effectors of innate immune system, NK-cells are able to recognize and directly kill foreign, senescent, transformed, and virus-infected cells [1]. Besides eliminating their targets, NK-cells modulate dendritic cell and T cell activity through cytokine and chemokine secretion. Recent results have also shown that NK-cells can kill activated T cells playing an immunoregulatory function [2, 3]. Due to their cytotoxic potential, their dependence on interleukin (IL)-15 and the expression of the transcription factor Eomes, NK-cells are classified into group 1 innate lymphoid cells [4].

NK-cells represent 10–15% of peripheral blood lymphocytes (PBL) and are characterized by surface expression of the CD56 neural cell adhesion molecule and lack of CD3 and CD19. Based on the level of CD56 expression, NK-cells have been further classified as $CD56^{bright}$, that account for about 10% of PBL NK-cells, and $CD56^{dim}$. The $CD56^{bright}$ and $-^{dim}$ NK-cell subsets are usually considered as functionally distinct, with predominant cytokine-secreting or cytotoxic activities, respectively. However, both subsets can share the same functions after stimulation [5].

$CD56^{bright}$ NK-cells are the most abundant in human tissues, particularly in case of inflammation or neoplastic transformation. Tissue-resident intrahepatic $CD56^{bright}$ NK-cells have been described, characterized by the expression of hallmarks such as CD69, chemokine receptors (CXCR6 and CCR5), and adhesion molecules [6].

E. Cariani
Toxicology and Advanced Diagnostics, Ospedale Civile S. Agostino-Estense, Modena, Italy

G. Missale (✉)
Laboratory of Viral Immunopathology, Unit of Infectious Diseases and Hepatology, Azienda Ospedaliero-Universitaria di Parma, Parma, Italy
e-mail: missale@tin.it

T.F. Greten (ed.), *Immunotherapy of Hepatocellular Carcinoma*,
DOI 10.1007/978-3-319-64958-0_2

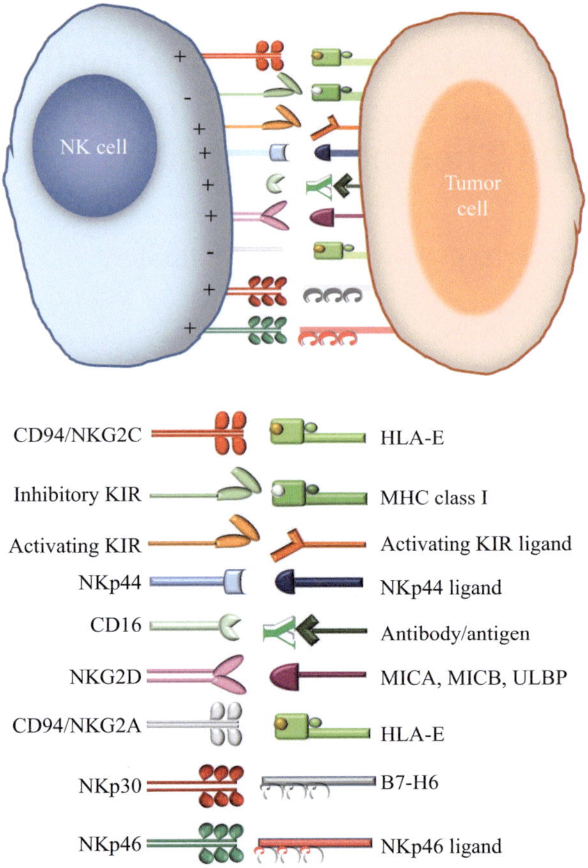

Fig. 2.1 Inhibitory and activating receptors expressed on the surface of NK cells. Inhibitory receptors recognize class I HLA ligands leading to inactivation of NK-cell function. The activation of NK anti-tumor effector function results from the down-regulation of self ligands and the expression of stress-induced ligands recognized by NK activating receptors

The distinct phenotype of tissue-resident NK-cells compared to their circulating counterpart is believed to reflect specific functional characteristics (reviewed in Ref. 7). CD56^{bright} NK-cells constitutively express high-affinity heterotrimeric IL-2 αβγ receptors, do not secrete IL-2 but, through release of other cytokines, i.e. interferon (IFN)-γ, play a major role in the regulation of the immune response [5].

The CD56^{dim} subset represents the large majority of circulating NK-cells and is far less abundant in tissues. Traditionally CD56^{dim} NK-cells are considered to differentiate from CD56^{bright} cells, however recent data indicate a wide phenotypic diversity, suggesting a more dynamic adjustment of NK-cell phenotype and function according to the genetic background and to the surrounding microenvironment [8].

The recognition of targets by NK-cells is driven by a complex system of surface receptors exerting either activating or inhibitory function (Fig. 2.1). Activating NK-cell receptors include the natural cytotoxicity receptors (NKp30, NKp44, NKp46), C-type lectin receptors NKG2D and CD94/NKG2C, CD16, and activating killer immunoglobulin-like receptors (KIRs), whereas inhibitory receptors include inhibitory KIRs and CD94/NKG2A heterodimer.

Tolerance is linked to the recognition of self major histocompatibility complex (MHC) class I by inhibitory KIRs and CD94/NKG2A. The recognition of MHC class I targets by inhibitory NK-cell receptors is also the basis of the process of licensing of immature NK-cells [9], and the down-regulation of MHC class I on transformed cells allows their identification by NK-cells.

The overall diversity of inhibitory NK-cell receptors, interacting with MHC class I ligands for maintenance of self tolerance, is strictly linked to the genetic background, whereas the expression of activating receptors is strongly influenced by environmental conditions [8]. Inhibitory signals usually overcome activating NK-cell receptors, that recognize stress-induced ligands expressed as a result of heat shock, viral infection, or genotoxic damage. Apart from receptor-ligand interactions, NK-cell activity is under the control of cytokines and of toll-like receptor ligands [10].

2.2 Alterations in NK-Cell Frequency, Phenotype and Function in Viral Hepatitis

The liver is directly exposed to the immune stimulation of gut-derived nutrients, bacteria and their metabolites. Tolerance to foreign antigens is maintained by liver-specific cell populations like Kupffer cells, liver sinusoidal endothelial cells (LSECs), hepatic stellate cells (HSCs) and even hepatocytes [11].

NK-cells represent 5–50% of intrahepatic immune infiltrate [12]. About 45% of the liver-infiltrating NK-cells consist of resident Eomes^{pos} CD56^{bright} NK-cells expressing CD69, CXCR6, CCR5 and NKp46, with low IFN-γ production and perforin and granzyme B expression [6].

NK-cells are primarily involved in response to virus and cancer. Hepatitis B (HBV) and C (HCV) viruses represent the main causes of liver disease worldwide and HCC is the most frequent complication of liver cirrhosis. It is then clear that understanding the interplay between NK-cells and hepatitis B and C viruses, is germane in order to define the role of NK-cells in the pathogenesis of HCC.

Several studies have addressed NK-cell phenotypic and functional modifications during HBV and HCV infection showing conflicting results for specific changes in different patients cohorts and experimental conditions, but agreeing in most cases on profound functional alteration of NK-cells. In most of the studies NK-cells are phenotypically activated with defect in cytokine (IFN-γ) production in HBV and HCV infected patients while cytotoxic function seems to be enhanced in patients with HCV infection.

Functional modification of NK-cell response in chronic HBV and HCV infection may be responsible for persistent inflammation in the liver, liver pathology, fibrosis due to NK-cell and HSC interaction and possibly to hepatocarcinogenesis because of inefficient surveillance by dysfunctional and/or exhausted NK-cells.

2.2.1 HBV

Chronic HBV infection has been associated with reduction of frequency as well as cytokine production of NK-cells compared to healthy controls. Several studies have reported a defect in IFN-γ production by NK-cells in patients with chronic hepatitis B [13–15], and mechanisms involved in downregulating NK-cell response may be represented by secretion of immunosuppressive cytokines such as IL-10 [16, 17]. Phenotypic modifications associated with functional alterations have been described with conflicting results. NKG2A was overexpressed with decreased cytotoxicity [18]. TIM-3, a co-inhibitor receptor, was overexpressed on peripheral and liver infiltrating NK-cells and blocking TIM-3 could restore IFN-γ production and cytotoxicity [19]. However, in two other studies [3, 17], cytotoxic granules and function were not different if compared with healthy subjects. A comparison of phenotypic and functional characteristics of circulating NK cells in patients with chronic HBV and HCV infection has shown lower frequency of activated NK cells in HBV infected patients with lower cytokine-induced cytolytic activity compared to subjects with chronic HCV infection [13].

Another mechanism played by NK-cells in patients with chronic HBV infection is killing of HBV-specific T cells by TNF-related apoptosis-inducing ligand (TRAIL)-TRAIL-R2 interaction [2], a regulatory function to limit T-cell mediated immunopathology. It is not known at this moment if similar mechanisms could negatively regulate tumor-specific T-cell response. Finally it is interesting to observe the behavior of NK-cells in patients undergoing antiviral treatment. Nucleoside analogs (NUCs) can efficiently block HBV replication, shutting down viral production with undetectable viremia, even though HBV can persist in its occult condition because of cccDNA mini chromosome that allows minimal levels of replication and antigen production. In patients undergoing NUC treatment with suppressed HBV replication, a reversion to a quiescent condition of NK-cells similar to healthy subjects has been observed. This was associated with reduced expression of TRAIL, CD38, and Ki67 and restoration of IFN-γ production [3].

2.2.2 HCV

Interplay between hepatitis C virus and NK-cells have been object of several studies. The first model was plate-bound HCV antigen E2 that could bind CD81, a tetraspanin expressed on epithelial and immune cells and in particular on NK-cells [20, 21]. This interaction was primarily shown to impair IFN-γ secretion. Later studies in HCV replicative in-vitro models [22, 23] or infected hepatoma cells [24], allowed NK-cells interaction with free viral particles. Results turned out quite different compared to plate-bound E2: no impairment of NK-cell function by interaction with soluble virions while direct contact with infected cells could downregulate NKG2D and NKp30 expression with impaired NK-cell function [24, 25]. However, in-vivo the interplay with accessory cells releasing interferons and cytokines may modify and overcome the inhibitory effect due to direct interaction with infected cells. Plasmacitoid dendritic cells can sense HCV and produce type I IFNs [26–29] with activating functional effect on NK-cells. Monocytes in presence of HCV can produce IL-18 and IL-10 with opposing effect on NK-cells cytokine production.

Studies conducted in chronically infected patients have shown that persistently activated NK-cells may be dysfunctional with reduced IFN-γ production because of exhaustion due to chronic persistent stimulation [30], while cytotoxic function resulted increased. This dichotomous condition has been ascribed to persistent exposure to IFN-α with STAT1 overexpression and phosphorylation that stimulates NK-cell cytotoxicity [31–34]. NKp46^{high} NK-cells are reported in the periphery and intrahepatic compartment of HCV infected patients [35] in agreement with enhanced cytotoxic potential. However other studies have underlined that even in presence of NKp46 upregulation in the liver, degranulation and TRAIL expression by intrahepatic NK-cells is reduced [36]. These apparently contrasting results may derive from differences in patients selection or by the fact that combined NKp46 expression with inhibitory receptor NKG2A is associated with reduced cytotoxicity as it has been shown in a previous study by our group in patients with HCV infection and HCC as well as in the uterine decidual NK-cells during pregnancy [37, 38].

Direct acting antivirals (DAAs) clear HCV within weeks of treatment in more than 90% of the cases. NK-cells can sense these changes with profound modification at phenotypic and functional levels. It has been shown that HCV clearance can determine phenotypic and functional effects on NK-cells in periphery and within the liver with durable reduced NK-cell activation associated with a rapid decline of NK-cell stimulating cytokines in serum such as IP-10, IL-12, IL-18 [39], providing an in-vivo model confirming the profound effect of HCV infection on NK-cell phenotype and function.

2.3 Alterations in NK Cell Frequency, Phenotype and Function in HCC

Previous data from patients with HCC showed a decreased NK subset in peripheral blood and a reduction in tumor-infiltrating NK-cells (especially the CD56^{dim}, CD16^{pos} subset) compared to the non-tumorous liver counterpart [40, 41]. Defective cytokine production and cytotoxic potential [40–43] were also described, mainly in advanced stage HCC [41]. NK-cell functional capacity was identified as a predictive factor for HCC outcome [42, 43].

In a recent study, the NK-cell dysfunction in patients with HCC has been related to a liver-infiltrating CD11b^{neg}CD27^{neg} NK-cell subset specifically increased in tumor tissue and showing both low cytotoxic and IFN-γ-secreting capacity. Enhanced multiplicity of CD11b^{neg}CD27^{neg} NK-cells was associated with advanced tumor stage, and represented a negative prognostic factor for survival [44].

Multiple molecular mechanisms linked to both genetic and environmental factors may be involved in shaping the NK-cell phenotype and function in HCC. In a recent study, we identified a relationship between better HCC prognosis and KIR2DS5, HLA-C1 and compound KIR2DL2-C1/KIR3DS1-Bw4I80 genotypes [45]. This relationship was supported by increased cytotoxic capacity of NK-cells from subjects with HLA-C1 alone or combined with KIR2DL2/KIR2DL3.

A genome-wide association study [46] identified an increased risk of HCC development in HCV patients with a single-nucleotide polymorphism in the gene encoding for MHC-associated chain A (MICA), a ligand of NKG2D. The MICA-NKG2D interaction had already been identified as a potential target of immune escape, since the proteolytic cleavage and shedding of soluble MICA (sMICA) in serum may induce down-regulation of NKG2D on NK-cell surface [47]. In patients with HCC elevated levels of sMICA were shown to be associated with decreased NKG2D expression and impaired NK cell activation [48]. In addition, decreased expression of the NKG2D ligand UL-16-binding protein (ULBP) 1 has been related to early recurrence of HCC after surgical resection [49].

A frequent mechanism driving functional impairment of NK-cells in solid tumors is the deregulated expression of the inhibitory receptor NKG2A and of its ligand, the non-classical MHC-I molecule HLA-E [50, 51]. This alteration may play a role in HCC, where HLA-E expression in hepatocytes is increased by the oncofetal protein Granulin – epithelin precursor, overexpressed in HCC [52]. We have recently observed a higher percentage of NK-cells co-expressing NKG2A, NKp30 and NKp46 in the peripheral blood of a subset of HCC patients with shorter survival [37]. This combined phenotype was negatively correlated to NK-cell function. Consistent with this observation, NKG2A co-engagement had previously been shown to inhibit NKp46-mediated cytotoxicity and NKp30-induced IFN-γ production in uterine decidual NK-cells during early pregnancy [38].

It is well known that the solid tumor microenvironment exerts a suppressive effect over immune response (Fig. 2.2). In particular, NK-cell phenotype is strongly influenced by cytokine concentration, presence of specific ligands for NK-cell receptors and infiltrating cell types. Both T regulatory cells (Tregs) and myeloid-derived suppressor cells (MDSCs) are key players in cancer immune evasion. Tregs are increased both in peripheral blood [53] and in tumor tissue [54] of patients with HCC, and enrichment of Tregs in tumor infiltrate is associated with disease progression and poor prognosis [55, 56].

A high prevalence of $CD14^{pos}$ $HLA\text{-}DR^{neg/low}$ MDSCs in tumor tissue and peripheral blood of patients with HCC was reported [57, 58]. MDSCs induce the expansion of Tregs through IL-10 and TGF-β production and impair hepatic NK-cell activity via membrane-bound TGF-β [59]. The direct inhibition of NK-cells by MDSCs *via* the activating receptor NKp30 has also been described in patients with HCC [43], and tumor monocytes have been shown to drive sequential activation and exhaustion/apoptosis of NK-cells through CD48/2B4 interaction [41].

Interestingly, a recent study showed that MDSCs recruited by senescent hepatocytes through CCL2-CCR2 signaling could prevent HCC initiation, but promoted progression of established HCC. In the HCC context MDSCs do not appear to

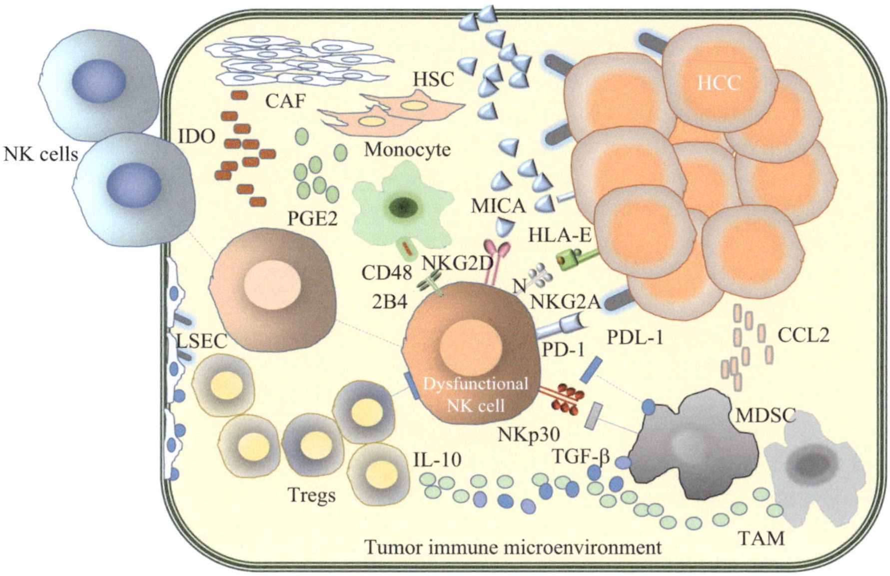

Fig. 2.2 Immune suppressive mechanisms of the HCC microenvironment. Intratumoral NK cell phenotype is shaped by cytokines, receptor-ligand interactions, tumor cells and infiltrating cells (mainly immature and suppressive cells). *CAF* cancer associated fibroblasts, *HSC* hepatic stellate cells, *PGE2* prostaglandin E-2, *IDO* indoleamine-2,3-dioxygenase

differentiate into macrophages, but accumulate creating an immunotolerant environment that enhances HCC growth by NK-cell inhibition, thus worsening the survival of HCC patients [60].

The HCC immune environment favors the polarization of macrophages to tumour-associated macrophages (TAMs), characterized by high IL-10 production that further induce Tregs expansion and impairs NK-cell activation [61].

Liver-resident cells are also involved in anti-tumor immune response. LSECs express PDL-1 and can induce Tregs in a TGF-β-dependent fashion [62]. HSCs contribute to MDSC and Treg induction [63, 64] and cancer-associated fibroblasts inhibit NK-cell function through the secretion of prostaglandin E2 and indoleamine-pyrrole 2,3-dioxygenase (IDO) [65].

2.4 Perspectives for NK-Cell-Based Immunotherapy in HCC

Immunotherapeutic strategies have long been focused on the activation of T cell response. However, more recently interest has been raised about the potential of NK-cells as therapeutic targets. Advantages of NK-cell-based treatment strategies include lack of antigen specificity, rapid acquisition of cytolytic function and enhanced killing activity towards cancer stem cells, a quiescent subset displaying increased tumorigenic potential and resistance to conventional therapies [66].

Although NK-cell-based strategies display enhanced efficacy in hematological malignancies [67], they hold potential for the treatment of solid tumors. Several approaches can be hypothesized to restore anti-tumor NK-cell function in the tumor microenvironment (reviewed in Ref. 68). Autologous or allogeneic NK-cells have been adoptively transferred after in vitro expansion by cytokines, although this approach did not lead to clinical response in advanced digestive tumors [69]. Cytokines can also be administered to expand NK-cells in vivo. IL-15 appears as the most promising agent in this context, since different from IL-2 it does not activate Tregs and has a stimulating effect on cytotoxic T lymphocytes. Adoptive NK-cell transfer, together with administration of IL-15 or of its superagonist ALT-803, is currently being tested in solid tumors [70]. The recent progress in knowledge of IL-15 signaling in NK-cells [71] discloses new perspectives for the genetic engineering of NK-cell function.

An attractive approach to enhance NK-cell anti-tumor activity is the targeting of surface receptors. Activating CD16 receptor co-operates in the therapeutic effect of tumor-targeting mAbs through the mechanism of antibody dependent cellular cytotoxicity (ADCC) [72], and this capacity is retained by adoptively transferred NK-cells. To further enhance NK-cell-mediated cytotoxicity, bi- and tri-specific antibodies have been designed able to bind both tumor antigens and an activating NK-cell receptor (e.g., CD16 or NKG2D) together with cytokines (e.g., IL-15). Several studies reported effective triggering of tumor cell lysis by the crosslinking of tumor and NK-cell targets (reviewed in Ref. 73).

Inhibitory NK-cell receptors represent another promising target: a recombinant anti-inhibitory KIRs monoclonal antibody (mAb) (Lirilumab, IPH2102) [74] is under evaluation both in hematological and solid tumors, as is monoalizumab (IPH2201), a blocking mAb to NKG2A.

Since the T cell checkpoint molecules CTLA-4 and PD-1 are also expressed by NK cells, the efficacy of anti-CTLA-4 and anti-PD-1/PDL-1 checkpoint inhibitors is at least partly linked to their influence on NK-cell function. Tim-3 is another potentially interesting checkpoint target for NK-cell-based immunotherapy. Tim-3 is upregulated on NK-cells from patients with solid tumors [75, 76] and blocking of Tim-3 appears to restore NK-cell activity [75]. Moreover, Tim-3 expression levels correlate with prognosis in gastric cancer [76] and in lung adenocarcinoma [77].

A novel and more versatile strategy is represented by BiKEs and TriKEs (Bi- and Tri-specific Killer cell Engagers), small molecules composed of 2–3 variable portions of antibodies with different specificities. BiKEs consist of 2 antibody fragments, recognizing a tumor antigen and CD16, respectively, that facilitate the formation of immunological synapses and trigger ADCC upon target recognition [78]. TriKEs integrate IL-15 in the above architecture, enhancing NK-cell expansion [79]. The TriKEs can be produced as recombinant proteins and used to stimulate endogenous NK-cells without the need for cell transfer, thus representing a flexible tool that can be customized to target different ligands and to bypass immunoediting of tumor-associated antigens (TAAs). Other activating NK-cell receptors (e.g., NKG2D) are potential candidates to be incorporated into recombinant immunotherapeutic tools [80]. However, further information is needed about the effect of these molecules on NK-cell function before their use in human therapy.

Combined therapies represent a promising strategy for treatment optimization. Drugs targeting the immunosuppressive tumor microenvironment (i.e., inhibitors of TGF-β or of adenosine receptor A2A) can be used to improve NK-cell function. In addition, anti-tumor drugs may display immunomodulatory effects targeting NK-cell function either directly (e.g., thalidomide, lenalidomide) or indirectly, by modulating the expression of NK-cell receptors or their ligands. These interactions may favor NK-cell function, as in the case of Sorafenib for the treatment of HCC [81], or alternatively be detrimental, supporting the need for careful evaluation of combined strategies.

Altogether, the results of NK-cell-targeted immunotherapeutic strategies in the context of HCC are still preliminary. Only part of the above described approaches have been employed to date and will be the main focus of the following paragraphs.

2.4.1 Adoptive Cell Transfer

The anti-tumor activity of autologous lymphokine-treated killer cells administered together with IL-2 was first reported in the 80s, but this approach was limited by side effects due to IL-2 toxicity and Treg-activating effect [82]. Since then, cytokine-induced killer cells (CIKs) have been frequently used for adoptive cell therapy in cancer patients. CIKs consist of activated T cells, activated NK-cells and NK T cells [83] and are usually obtained *ex vivo* from PBMCs stimulated by cytokines (IFN-γ, IL-2) and anti-CD3 antibodies. The anti-tumor immune response of CIKs appears to rely on the interaction between NKG2D and its ligands MICA and -B [84]. Safety of CIK therapy in HCC was reported in two single-arm, prospective studies [85, 86]. Two randomized controlled trials [87, 88] evaluated adjuvant CIK therapy after surgical resection of HCC, showing improved recurrence-free survival but no effect on overall survival, in contrast to a retrospective study reporting a survival advantage of CIK-treated patients [89]. CIK administration together with or after loco-regional treatments was also shown to increase progression-free survival, overall survival or both in randomized and retrospective studies [90–92]. The efficacy and safety of CIK injections as adjuvant therapy after curative treatment of HCC was also recently evaluated in a multicenter, randomized, open-label, phase III trial. Results showed increased recurrence-free and overall survival without difference in the rate of serious adverse events compared to patients not receiving immunotherapy [93].

2.4.2 Monoclonal Antibodies (mAbs)

Different mAb-based immunotherapeutic strategies can be used for the restoration of anti-tumor NK-cell function. Activating and co-stimulatory NK-cell receptors can be triggered by agonistic mAbs, and inhibitory NK receptors can be blocked by mAbs to release NK-cell function. To date these approaches have had limited application in HCC although they may represent possible tools for combined immunotherapeutic strategies. Targeting of checkpoint molecules expressed by different cell subsets represents a more promising therapeutic tool. The use of mAbs against CTLA-4, PD-1 or its ligand PDL-1 have been a major breakthrough in the treatment of several types of cancer [94]. Although these checkpoint inhibitors are believed to exert their main effect through their influence on T cell activity, they also contribute to restore anti-tumor NK-cell function.

CTLA-4 is expressed on activated T cells and Tregs [95]. CTLA-4 antagonizes the CD28 binding to CD80 and CD86 [96] thus inhibiting T-cell activation. Experimental evidence has revealed that the anti-tumor activity of CTLA-4 blockade results from effects on both effector T cells and Treg cells, that are eliminated by a NK-cell and macrophage-dependent ADCC mechanism [97]. As a consequence, suppression of CTLA-4 function may result in non-antigen specific autoimmune phenotypes [98].

The anti-CTLA-4 mAb Tremelimumab, belonging to the IgG2 subclass, was tested by a pilot trial in 21 patients with inoperable HCC and chronic HCV infection showing a good safety profile, despite transient but intense elevations of transaminase levels after the first dose in 45% of patients. Despite modest anti-tumor effect (partial response rate: 17.6%, disease control rate: 76.4%, time to progression: 6.4 months), anti-viral activity was reported, with decreased viral load, development of anti-HCV immune responses and emergence of new viral variants [99]. Although the results of this study did not provide a definitive proof of anti-tumor efficacy, they offered a rationale for immune checkpoint inhibition in HCC. Trememlimumab administration before ablative treatment was recently tested in advanced HCC. Of 19/32 patients evaluable, 5 had a partial response with increase in intratumoral $CD8^{pos}$ T cells. A marked reduction in HCV RNA load was also observed in 12/14 patients. Median time to tumor progression was 7.4 months and median OS 12.3 months [100].

PD-1 is expressed in different cell populations, including T, B, and myeloid cells [101]. Recently, high PD-1 expression was shown in a subset of peripheral blood $CD56^{dim}NKG2A^{neg}KIR^{pos}CD57^{pos}$ NK-cells both in healthy donors and, more frequently, in patients with ovarian carcinoma with enrichment in the ascitic fluid, suggesting the induction of this cell population in the tumor microenvironment. This $PD\text{-}1^{pos}$ NK-cell subset displayed impaired degranulation/cytotoxic activity that could be rescued by anti–PDL antibodies in vitro [102]. These data offer a rationale for PD-1-PDL-1 pathway blockade to restore anti-tumor NK-cell function.

Variable levels of PDL-1 expression have been reported in HCC [54, 103, 104]. Immunostaining with anti-PDL-1 antibodies suggested a preferential localization in tumor cells compared to infiltrating lymphomononuclear cells and stromal cell elements [54]. In addition, PDL-1 expression levels appear to be related to overall survival of HCC patients [54, 103, 104] thus supporting the relevance of the PD-1-PDL-1 pathway in the impaired immune surveillance of HCC.

The safety and antitumor effect of Nivolumab, a fully human IgG4 anti-PD-1 mAb was evaluated in patients with advanced HCC virus-related or non-virus-related, by an international multicentre phase I/II trial started in 2012 [105]. Both patients exposed or not exposed to the kinase inhibitor sorafenib were enrolled, showing acceptable safety profile and durable responses. A human IgG1 anti-PDL-1 mAb, MED14736, has also demonstrated activity in solid tumors including HCC [106].

Anti-tumor NK-cell function may be triggered by antibodies against TAAs driving NK-cell ADCC of tumor cells. A recent randomized phase II trial tested Codrituzumab, a humanized monoclonal antibody against Glypican-3 (GPC3) that is expressed in HCC, vs. placebo in advanced HCC patients who had failed prior systemic therapy. Codrituzumab treatment had an adverse event profile identical to placebo, but did not show clinical benefit. However, results suggested that a higher dose of codrituzumab or the selection of patients with high level of GPC3 or CD16 might improve outcome [107].

2.4.3 *Genetically Modified NK*

NK-cells can be engineered to improve their in vivo persistence, expansion potential, and tumor targeting capacity. To date, immunotherapeutic approaches involving the use of genetically modified NK-cells have not been applied to HCC but they represent an interesting perspective for future clinical applications.

IL-2 gene delivery in expanded NK-cells [108] and genetic manipulation of NK-cells for ectopic expression of IL-15 [109] have been used to enhance NK-cell function. Introduction of genes to induce resistance to suppressive cytokines has also been proposed to enhance NK-cell cytotoxic capacity. Adoptive transfer of a NK-92 cell line expressing the dominant negative mutant form of TGFβ type II receptor (DNTβRII) on their surface was shown to increase survival in lung-cancer bearing mice compared to wild-type NK-92 [110].

NK-cells can be engineered by the insertion of chimeric antigen receptors (CARs) that provide specificity towards a tumor antigen triggering NK-cell cytotoxicity upon target recognition. CARs include an extracellular domain (generally a small chain variable fragment) specific for a tumor antigen, and one or more intracellular domains able to induce activation signals. It has been shown that CAR-expressing NK-cells are able to elicit a stronger cytolytic response compared to ADCC [111].

CAR-bearing NK-cells display several potential advantages compared to T cells. Since CAR-transduced NK-cells are more short-lived than their T cell counterparts and do not express autocrine growth factors (i.e., IL-2), they do not need “suicide genes” to limit the risk of autoimmune reaction. Furthermore, the cytokine profile of NK-cells is less prone to induce severe adverse reactions compared to CAR-expressing T cells [112]. Finally, NK-cell cytotoxicity can be triggered by several activating receptors even in the event of target antigen loss by the tumor. However, one major drawback for the generation of CAR-NK is the difficulty of isolating and expanding NK-cells, that could be overcome by the use of NK-cell lines (e.g., NK-92), easier to expand and to engineer.

2.4.4 Combined Approaches

NK-cell response is inefficient controlling HCC. This is the result of tumor microenvironment acting through different possible mechanisms, but it may be also due to resistance of tumor cells to NK cytotoxic response. This may be due to insufficient exposure of NK ligands on target cells, release of soluble mediators preventing interaction between NK and tumor cell or intrinsic resistance of target cells to apoptosis.

High serum levels of sMICA binding NKG2D and preventing recognition of its ligands on HCC is one possible mechanisms of target escape that has been suggested for HCV-related hepatocellular carcinoma by genome wide association studies that showed increased HCC occurrence in HCV patients presenting the MICA variant, rs23596542 responsible of high serum levels of sMICA [113].

Making HCC more susceptible to NK cytotoxic response may represent a relevant strategy to treat hepatocellular carcinoma. Anti-tumor agents already tested in HCC patients and new molecules under study could potentiate adoptive immunotherapeutic approaches like adoptive transfer of activated NK-cells or other NK-cell mediated immunotherapies.

Sorafenib, the multikinase inhibitor that represents standard of care for patients with advanced HCC, has been shown to induce a decline of the metalloprotease ADAM9 that is usually upregulated in human HCC [114]. ADAM family metalloproteases have been shown to be responsible for proteolytic release of the ectodomain of transmembranous proteins like MICA. Even if this is a preclinical study, ADAM9 is also overexpressed in HCC patients suggesting that sorafenib effect could in part be due by an indirect mechanism linked to enhanced NK-cell response. However other studies have pointed out that sorafenib, affecting PI3K and ERK phosphorylation, may exert a direct inhibitory effect on NK-cell response [115]. Definitive studies on the real effect of sorafenib on the anti-tumor immune response in-vivo and in particular on the NK-cell response are still lacking, so at present we have to be cautious on the possible combined use of sorafenib and immunotherapeutic treatments.

Modulation of NKG2D targets on tumor cells have been addressed by studies focused on histone deacetylase inhibitors (HDACIs) that can induce expression of MICA on HCC cells in-vitro. These molecules have been tested in-vivo in solid tumors and also in patients with HCC showing good safety profile and high rate of tumor stabilization [116]. In a recent study a library of 636 FDA-approved drugs was screened in order to identify the most effective molecules in promoting MICA expression in HCC. The search identified the HDACI Vorinostat as the candidate molecule [117] able to significantly increase NK-cell mediated HCC cytotoxicity *in vitro*. The cytotoxic effect was further enhanced by the combined use of inhibitors of MICA shedding.

Another mechanism to boost NK-cell cytotoxic response is down regulation of HLA-class I, thus reducing the inhibitory signal provided by KIR-HLA binding. Bortezomib, a cancer drug that has been tested in several tumors but in particular in patients with multiple myeloma, has been shown to sensitize tumor cells to NK-cell cytotoxicity by down regulation of HLA-class I and also by up regulation of ligands for NK-cell activating receptors like TNF receptor apoptosis-related protein p55 (TNFRp55) and molecules of the death receptor (DR) family [118]. To date bortezomib effect, sensitizing HCC to NK-cell response, has been demonstrated in a preclinical HCC model [119] by upregulation of NKG2DL and ULBP families with increased NK-cell response, but its effect *in vivo* has not been confirmed yet.

In conclusion several anti-tumor drugs may sensitize target tumor cells favoring NK-cell response and this may represent a synergic mechanism of action to be exploited for combined immunotherapeutic approaches.

2.5 Conclusions

Despite developing in a context of chronic inflammation, HCC is surrounded by an immunosuppressive microenvironment. Tumor-infiltrating immune cells are dysfunctional but their cytotoxic potential can be restored *in vitro* and *in vivo*. Due to their functional characteristics, NK-cells represent promising therapeutic targets, but their complex biology hampers the development of appropriate immunotherapeutic strategies. The co-existence of regulatory and cytotoxic functions, exerted by licensed and non-licensed cell subsets, should not be overlooked in view of possible adverse effects. In addition, a deeper knowledge of NK-cell homing mechanisms will be instrumental to improve the results obtained in the treatment of solid tumors.

Several issues should also be addressed concerning the specific context of HCC. The influence of liver tissue immune *milieu* that likely plays a major role over the functional status of NK-cells has to be considered in order to enhance their functional capacity. The anti-tumor effect of NK-cell-based strategies should be optimized by integration with other immunotherapeutic approaches, targeted systemic therapies, ablative and loco-regional treatments, the last potentially able to synergize with immune therapies. Safety concerns linked to hepatotoxicity or to possible reactivation of hepatitis virus infections should also be considered. Finally, biomarkers should be developed to identify patients that may benefit from treatment and to limit the incidence of adverse effects.

The encouraging results of the first attempts to bring the NK-cell based immunotherapeutic approaches into the clinic pave the way towards a wider application in the treatment of HCC and, hopefully, towards prognostic improvements.

References

1. Vivier E, Tomasello E, Baratin M, Walzer T, Ugolini S. Functions of natural killer cells. Nat Immunol. 2008;9:503–10.
2. Peppa D, Gill US, Reynolds G, Easom NJ, Pallett LJ, Schurich A, et al. Up-regulation of a death receptor renders antiviral T cells susceptible to NK cell-mediated deletion. J Exp Med. 2013;21:99–114.

3. Boni C, Lampertico P, Talamona L, Giuberti T, Invernizzi F, Barili V, et al. Natural killer cell phenotype modulation and natural killer/T-cell interplay in nucleos(t)ide analogue-treated hepatitis e antigen-negative patients with chronic hepatitis B. Hepatology. 2015;62:1697–709.
4. Spits H, Artis D, Colonna M, Diefenbach A, Di Santo JP, Eberl G, et al. Innate lymphoid cells – a proposal for uniform nomenclature. Nat Rev Immunol. 2013;13:145–9.
5. Michel T, Poli A, Cuapio A, Briquemont B, Iserentant G, Ollert M, et al. Human CD56bright NK Cells: An Update. J Immunol. 2016;196:2923–31.
6. Stegmann KA, Robertson F, Hansi N, Gill U, Pallant C, Christophides T, et al. CXCR6 marks a novel subset of T-bet(lo)Eomes(hi) natural killer cells residing in human liver. Sci Rep. 2016;6:26157.
7. Melsen JE, Lugthart G, Lankester AC, Schilham MW. Human Circulating and Tissue-Resident CD56(bright) Natural Killer Cell Populations. Front Immunol. 2016;7:262.
8. Horowitz A, Strauss-Albee DM, Leipold M, Kubo J, Nemat-Gorgani N, Dogan OC, et al. Genetic and environmental determinants of human NK cell diversity revealed by mass cytometry. Sci Transl Med. 2013;5:208ra145.
9. Höglund P, Brodin P. Current perspectives of natural killer cell education by MHC class I molecules. Nat Rev Immunol. 2010;10:724–34.
10. Heymann F, Tacke F. Immunology in the liver – from homeostasis to disease. Nat Rev Gastroenterol Hepatol. 2016;13:88–110.
11. Thomson AW, Knolle PA. Antigen-presenting cell function in the tolerogenic liver environment. Nat Rev Immunol. 2010;10:753–66.
12. Gao B, Jeong WI, Tian Z. Liver: an organ with predominant innate immunity. Hepatology. 2008;47:729–36.
13. Oliviero B, Varchetta S, Paudice E, Michelone G, Zaramella M, Mavilio D, et al. Natural killer cell functional dichotomy in chronic hepatitis B and chronic hepatitis C virus infections. Gastroenterology. 2009;137:1151–60.
14. Peppa D, Micco L, Javaid A, Kennedy PT, Schurich A, Dunn C, et al. Blockade of immunosuppressive cytokines restores NK cell antiviral function in chronic hepatitis B virus infection. PLoS Pathog. 2010;6:e1001227.
15. Tjwa ET, van Oord GW, Hegmans JP, Janssen HL, Woltman AM. Viral load reduction improves activation and function of natural killer cells in patients with chronic hepatitis B. J Hepatol. 2011;54:209–18.
16. Harada N, Shimada M, Okano S, Suehiro T, Soejima Y, Tomita Y, et al. IL-12 gene therapy is an effective therapeutic strategy for hepatocellular carcinoma in immunosuppressed mice. J Immunol. 2004;173:6635–44.
17. Gonzalez-Carmona MA, Lukacs-Kornek V, Timmerman A, Shabani S, Kornek M, Vogt A, et al. CD40 ligand expressing dendritic cells induce regression of hepatocellular carcinoma by activating innate and acquired immunity in vivo. Hepatology. 2008;48:157–68.
18. Hato T, Goyal L, Greten TF, Duda D, Zhu A. Immune checkpoint blockade in hepatocellular carcinoma: current progress and future directions. Hepatology. 2014;60:1776–82.
19. Ju Y, Hou N, Meng J, Wang X, Zhang X, et al. T cell immunoglobulin- and mucin-domain-containing molecule-3 (Tim-3) mediates natural killer cell suppression in chronic hepatitis B. J Hepatol. 2010;52:322–9.
20. Crotta S, Stilla A, Wack A, D'Andrea A, Nuti S, D'Oro U, et al. Inhibition of natural killer cells through engagement of CD81 by the major hepatitis C virus envelope protein. J Exp Med. 2002;195:35–41.
21. Tseng CT, Klimpel GR. Binding of the hepatitis C virus envelope protein E2 to CD81 inhibits natural killer cell functions. J Exp Med. 2002;195:43–9.
22. Crotta S, Brazzoli M, Piccioli D, Valiante NM, Wack A. Hepatitis C virions subvert natural killer cell activation to generate a cytokine environment permissive for infection. J Hepatol. 2010;52:183–90.
23. Yoon JC, Shiina M, Ahlenstiel G, Rehermann B. Natural killer cell function is intact after direct exposure to infectious hepatitis C virions. Hepatology. 2009;49(1):12–21.

24. Yoon JC, Lim JB, Park JH, Lee JM. Cell-to-cell contact with hepatitis C virus-infected cells reduces functional capacity of natural killer cells. J Virol. 2011;85:12557–69.
25. Holder KA, Stapleton SN, Gallant ME, Russell RS, Grant MD. Hepatitis C virus-infected cells downregulate NKp30 and inhibit ex vivo NK cell functions. J Immunol. 2013;191:3308–18.
26. Dental C, Florentin J, Aouar B, Gondois-Rey F, Durantel D, Baumert TF, et al. Hepatitis C virus fails to activate NF-| B signaling in plasmacytoid dendritic cells. J Virol. 2012;86:1090–6.
27. Takahashi K, Asabe S, Wieland S, Garaigorta U, Gastaminza P, Isogawa M, et al. Plasmacytoid dendritic cells sense hepatitis C virus-infected cells, produce interferon, and inhibit infection. Proc Natl Acad Sci U S A. 2010;107:7431–6.
28. Zhang XA, Huang C. Tetraspanins and cell membrane tubular structures. Cell Mol Life Sci. 2012;69:2843–52.
29. Dreux M, Garaigorta U, Boyd B, Décembre E, Chung J, Whitten-Bauer C, et al. Short-range exosomal transfer of viral RNA from infected cells to plasmacytoid dendritic cells triggers innate immunity. Cell Host Microbe. 2012;12:558–70.
30. Park SH, Rehermann B. Immune responses to HCV and other hepatitis viruses. Immunity. 2014;40:13–24.
31. Edlich B, Ahlenstiel G, Zabaleta Azpiroz A, Stoltzfus J, Noureddin M, Serti E, et al. Early changes in interferon signaling define natural killer cell response and refractoriness to interferon-based therapy of hepatitis C patients. Hepatology. 2012;55:39–48.
32. Miyagi T, Gil MP, Wang X, Louten J, Chu WM, Biron CA. High basal STAT4 balanced by STAT1 induction to control type 1 interferon effects in natural killer cells. J Exp Med. 2007;204:2383–96.
33. Miyagi T, Takehara T, Nishio K, Shimizu S, Kohga K, Li W, et al. Altered interferon-alpha-signaling in natural killer cells from patients with chronic hepatitis C virus infection. J Hepatol. 2010;53:424–30.
34. Nguyen KB, Cousens LP, Doughty LA, Pien GC, Durbin JE, Biron CA. Interferon alpha/beta-mediated inhibition and promotion of interferon gamma: STAT1 resolves a paradox. Nat Immunol. 2000;1:70–6.
35. Ahlenstiel G, Titerence RH, Koh C, Edlich B, Feld JJ, Rotman Y, et al. Natural killer cells are polarized toward cytotoxicity in chronic hepatitis C in an interferon-alfa-dependent manner. Gastroenterology. 2010;138:325–35.
36. Varchetta S, Mele D, Mantovani S, Oliviero B, Cremonesi E, Ludovisi S, et al. Impaired intrahepatic natural killer cell cytotoxic function in chronic hepatitis C virus infection. Hepatology. 2012;56:841–9.
37. Cariani E, Pilli M, Barili V, Porro E, Biasini E, Olivani A, et al. Natural killer cells phenotypic characterization as an outcome predictor of HCV-linked HCC after curative treatments. Oncoimmunology. 2016;5:e1154249.
38. El Costa H, Casemayou A, Aguerre-Girr M, Rabot M, Berrebi A, Parant O, et al. Critical and differential roles of NKp46- and NKp30-activating receptors expressed by uterine NK cells in early pregnancy. J Immunol. 2008;181:3009–17.
39. Serti E, Chepa-Lotrea X, Kim YJ, Keane M, Fryzek N, Liang TJ, et al. Successful interferon-free therapy of chronic hepatitis C virus infection normalizes natural killer cell function. Gastroenterology. 2015;149:190–200.
40. Cai L, Zhang Z, Zhou L, Wang H, Fu J, Zhang S, et al. Functional impairment in circulating and intrahepatic NK cells and relative mechanism in hepatocellular carcinoma patients. Clin Immunol. 2008;129:428–37.
41. Wu Y, Kuang DM, Pan WD, Wan YL, Lao XM, Wang D, et al. Monocyte/macrophage-elicited natural killer cell dysfunction in hepatocellular carcinoma is mediated by CD48/2B4 interactions. Hepatology. 2013;57:1107–16.
42. Taketomi A, Shimada M, Shirabe K, Kajiyama K, Gion T, Sugimachi K. Natural killer cell activity in patients with hepatocellular carcinoma: a new prognostic indicator after hepatectomy. Cancer. 1998;83:58–63.

43. Hoechst B, Voigtlaender T, Ormandy L, Gamrekelashvili J, Zhao F, Wedemeyer H, et al. Myeloid derived suppressor cells inhibit natural killer cells in patients with hepatocellular carcinoma via the NKp30 receptor. Hepatology. 2009;50:799–807.
44. Zhang QF, Yin WW, Xia Y, Yi YY, He QF, Wang X, et al. Liver-infiltrating CD11b(−)CD27(−) NK subsets account for NK-cell dysfunction in patients with hepatocellular carcinoma and are associated with tumor progression. Cell Mol Immunol. 2016; doi:10.1038/cmi.2016.28. [Epub ahead of print]
45. Cariani E, Pilli M, Zerbini A, Rota C, Olivani A, Zanelli P, et al. HLA and killer immunoglobulin-like receptor genes as outcome predictors of hepatitis C virus-related hepatocellular carcinoma. Clin Cancer Res. 2013;19:5465–73.
46. Kumar V, Kato N, Urabe Y, Takahashi A, Muroyama R, Hosono N, et al. Genome-wide association study identifies a susceptibility locus for HCV-induced hepatocellular carcinoma. Nat Genet. 2011;43:455–8.
47. Groh V, Wu J, Yee C, Spies T. Tumour-derived soluble MIC ligands impair expression of NKG2D and T-cell activation. Nature. 2002;419:734–8.
48. Jinushi M, Takehara T, Tatsumi T, Hiramatsu N, Sakamori R, Yamaguchi S, et al. Impairment of natural killer cell and dendritic cell functions by the soluble form of MHC class I-related chain A in advanced human hepatocellular carcinomas. J Hepatol. 2005;43:1013–20.
49. Kamimura H, Yamagiwa S, Tsuchiya A, Takamura M, Matsuda Y, Ohkoshi S, et al. Reduced NKG2D ligand expression in hepatocellular carcinoma correlates with early recurrence. J Hepatol. 2012;56:381–8.
50. Mamessier E, Sylvain A, Thibult ML, Houvenaeghel G, Jacquemier J, Castellano R, et al. Human breast cancer cells enhance self tolerance by promoting evasion from NK cell antitumor immunity. J Clin Invest. 2011;121:3609–22.
51. Bossard C, Bezieau S, Matysiak-Budnik T, Volteau C, Laboisse CL, Jotereau F, et al. HLA-E/β2 microglobulin overexpression in colorectal cancer is associated with recruitment of inhibitory immune cells and tumor progression. Int J Cancer. 2012;131:855–63.
52. Cheung PF, Yip CW, Wong NC, Fong DY, Ng LW, Wan AM, et al. Granulin-epithelin precursor renders hepatocellular carcinoma cells resistant to natural killer cytotoxicity. Cancer Immunol Res. 2014;2:1209–19.
53. Ormandy LA, Hillemann T, Wedemeyer H, Manns MP, Greten TF, Korangy F. Increased populations of regulatory T cells in peripheral blood of patients with hepatocellular carcinoma. Cancer Res. 2005;65:2457–64.
54. Cariani E, Pilli M, Zerbini A, Rota C, Olivani A, Pelosi G, et al. Immunological and molecular correlates of disease recurrence after liver resection for hepatocellular carcinoma. PLoS One. 2012;7:e32493.
55. Gao Q, Qiu SJ, Fan J, Zhou J, Wang XY, Xiao YS, et al. Intratumoral balance of regulatory and cytotoxic T cells is associated with prognosis of hepatocellular carcinoma after resection. J Clin Oncol. 2007;25:2586–93.
56. Chen KJ, Lin SZ, Zhou L, Xie HY, Zhou WH, Taki-Eldin A, et al. Selective recruitment of regulatory T cell through CCR6-CCL20 in hepatocellular carcinoma fosters tumor progression and predicts poor prognosis. PLoS One. 2011;6:e24671.
57. Hoechst B, Ormandy LA, Ballmaier M, Lehner F, Krüger C, Manns MP, et al. A new population of myeloid derived suppressor cells in hepatocellular carcinoma patients induces CD4(+)CD25(+)Foxp3(+) T cells. Gastroenterology. 2008;135:234–43.
58. Arihara F, Mizukoshi E, Kitahara M, Takata Y, Arai K, Yamashita T, et al. Increase in CD14+HLA-DR −/low myeloid-derived suppressor cells in hepatocellular carcinoma patients and its impact on prognosis. Cancer Immunol Immunother. 2013;62:1421–30.
59. Li H, Han Y, Guo Q, Zhang M, Cao X. Cancer-expanded myeloid-derived suppressor cells induce anergy of NK cells through membrane-bound TGF-β1. J Immunol. 2009;182:240–9.
60. Eggert T, Wolter K, Ji J, Ma C, Yevsa T, Klotz S, et al. Distinct functions of senescence-associated immune responses in liver tumor surveillance and tumor progression. Cancer Cell. 2016;30:533–47.

61. Ostrand-Rosenberg S, Sinha P, Beury DW, Ma C, Yevsa T, Klotz S, et al. Cross-talk between myeloid-derived suppressor cells (MDSC), macrophages, and dendritic cells enhances tumor-induced immune suppression. Semin Cancer Biol. 2012;22:275–81.
62. Carambia A, Freund B, Schwinge D, Heine M, Laschtowitz A, Huber S, et al. TGF-β-dependent induction of CD4+CD25+Foxp3+ Tregs by liver sinusoidal endothelial cells. J Hepatol. 2014;61:594–9.
63. Dunham RM, Thapa M, Velazquez VM, Elrod EJ, Denning TL, Pulendran B, et al. Hepatic stellate cells preferentially induce Foxp3+ regulatory T cells by production of retinoic acid. J Immunol. 2013;190:2009–16.
64. Höchst B, Schildberg FA, Sauerborn P, Gäbel YA, Gevensleben H, Goltz D, et al. Activated human hepatic stellate cells induce myeloid derived suppressor cells from peripheral blood monocytes in a CD44-dependent fashion. J Hepatol. 2013;59:528–35.
65. Li T, Yang Y, Hua X, Wang G, Liu W, Jia C, et al. Hepatocellular carcinoma-associated fibroblasts trigger NK cell dysfunction via PGE2 and IDO. Cancer Lett. 2012;318:154–61.
66. Grossenbacher SK, Canter RJ, Murphy WJ. Natural killer cell immunotherapy to target stem-like tumor cells. J Immunother Cancer. 2016;4:19.
67. Ruggeri L, Capanni M, Urbani E, Perruccio K, Shlomchik WD, Tosti A, et al. Effectiveness of donor natural killer cell alloreactivity in mismatched hematopoietic transplants. Science. 2002;295:2097–100.
68. Guillerey C, Huntington ND, Smyth MJ. Targeting natural killer cells in cancer immunotherapy. Nat Immunol. 2016;17:1025–36.
69. Sakamoto N, Ishikawa T, Kokura S, Okayama T, Oka K, Ideno M, et al. Phase I clinical trial of autologous NK cell therapy using novel expansion method in patients with advanced digestive cancer. J Transl Med. 2015;13:277.
70. Kim PS, Kwilas AR, Xu W, Alter S, Jeng EK, Wong HC, et al. IL-15 superagonist/IL-15RαSushi-Fc fusion complex (IL-15SA/IL-15RαSu-Fc; ALT-803) markedly enhances specific subpopulations of NK and memory CD8+ T cells, and mediates potent anti-tumor activity against murine breast and colon carcinomas. Oncotarget. 2016;7:16130–45.
71. Delconte RB, Kolesnik TB, Dagley LF, Rautela J, Shi W, Putz EM, et al. CIS is a potent checkpoint in NK cell-mediated tumor immunity. Nat Immunol. 2016;17:816–24.
72. Weng WK, Levy R. Two immunoglobulin G fragment C receptor polymorphisms independently predict response to rituximab in patients with follicular lymphoma. J Clin Oncol. 2003;21:3940–7.
73. Morvan MG, Lanier LL. NK cells and cancer: you can teach innate cells new tricks. Nat Rev Cancer. 2016;16:7–19.
74. Kohrt HE, Thielens A, Marabelle A, Sagiv-Barfi I, Sola C, Chanuc F, et al. Anti-KIR antibody enhancement of anti-lymphoma activity of natural killer cells as monotherapy and in combination with anti-CD20 antibodies. Blood. 2014;123:678–86.
75. da Silva IP, Gallois A, Jimenez-Baranda S, Khan S, Anderson AC, Kuchroo VK, et al. Reversal of NK-cell exhaustion in advanced melanoma by Tim-3 blockade. Cancer Immunol Res. 2014;2:410–22.
76. Wang Z, Zhu J, Gu H, Yuan Y, Zhang B, Zhu D, et al. The clinical significance of abnormal Tim-3 expression on NK cells from patients with gastric cancer. Immunol Investig. 2015;44:578–89.
77. Xu L, Huang Y, Tan L, Yu W, Chen D, Lu C, et al. Increased Tim-3 expression in peripheral NK cells predicts a poorer prognosis and Tim-3 blockade improves NK cell-mediated cytotoxicity in human lung adenocarcinoma. Int Immunopharmacol. 2015;29:635–41.
78. Gleason MK, Ross JA, Warlick ED, Lund TC, Verneris MR, Wiernik A, et al. CD16xCD33 bispecific killer cell engager (BiKE) activates NK cells against primary MDS and MDSC CD33C targets. Blood. 2014;123:3016–26.
79. Vallera DA, Felices M, McElmurry RT, McCullar V, Zhou X, Schmohl JU, et al. IL-15 Trispecific Killer Engagers (TriKEs) make natural killer cells specific to CD33+ targets

while also inducing persistence, in vivo expansion, and enhanced function. Clin Cancer Res. 2016;22:3440–50.
80. Tay SS, Carol H, Biro M. TriKEs and BiKEs join CARs on the cancer immunotherapy highway. Hum Vaccin Immunother. 2016;12:2790–6.
81. Sprinzl MF, Reisinger F, Puschnik A, Ringelhan M, Ackermann K, Hartmann D, et al. Sorafenib perpetuates cellular anticancer effector functions by modulating the crosstalk between macrophages and natural killer cells. Hepatology. 2013;57:2358–68.
82. Rosenberg SA, Lotze MT, Muul LM, Leitman S, Chang AE, Ettinghausen SE, et al. Observations on the systemic administration of autologous lymphokine-activated killer cells and recombinant interleukin-2 to patients with metastatic cancer. N Engl J Med. 1985;313:1485–92.
83. Zoll B, Lefterova P, Csipai M, Finke S, Trojaneck B, Ebert O, et al. Generation of cytokine-induced killer cells using exogenous interleukin-2, −7 or −12. Cancer Immunol Immunother. 1998;47:221–6.
84. Morisaki T, Hirano T, Koya N, Kiyota A, Tanaka H, Umebayashi M, et al. NKG2D-directed cytokine-activated killer lymphocyte therapy combined with gemcitabine for patients with chemoresistant metastatic solid tumors. Anticancer Res. 2014;34:4529–38.
85. Shi M, Zhang B, Tang ZR, Lei ZY, Wang HF, Feng YY, et al. Autologous cytokine-induced killer cell therapy in clinical trial Phase I is safe in patients with primary hepatocellular carcinoma. World J Gastroenterol. 2004;10:1146–51.
86. Ma H, Zhang Y, Wang Q, Li Y, He J, Wang H, et al. Therapeutic safety and effects of adjuvant autologous RetroNectin activated killer cell immunotherapy for patients with primary hepatocellular carcinoma after radiofrequency ablation. Cancer Biol Ther. 2010;9:903–7.
87. Takayama T, Sekine T, Makuuchi M, Yamasaki S, Kosuge T, Yamamoto J, et al. Adoptive immunotherapy to lower postsurgical recurrence rates of hepatocellular carcinoma: a randomised trial. Lancet. 2000;356:802–7.
88. Hui D, Qiang L, Jian W, Ti Z, Da-Lu K. A randomized, controlled trial of postoperative adjuvant cytokine-induced killer cells immunotherapy after radical resection of hepatocellular carcinoma. Dig Liver Dis. 2009;41:36–41.
89. Pan K, Li YQ, Wang W, Xu L, Zhang YJ, Zheng HX, et al. The efficacy of cytokine-induced killer cell infusion as an adjuvant therapy for postoperative hepatocellular carcinoma patients. Ann Surg Oncol. 2013;20:4305–11.
90. Weng DS, Zhou J, Zhou QM, Zhao M, Wang QJ, Huang LX, et al. Minimally invasive treatment combined with cytokine-induced killer cells therapy lower the short-term recurrence rates of hepatocellular carcinomas. J Immunother. 2008;31:63–71.
91. Huang ZM, Li W, Li S, Gao F, Zhou QM, Wu FM, et al. Cytokine-induced killer cells in combination with transcatheter arterial chemoembolization and radiofrequency ablation for hepatocellular carcinoma patients. J Immunother. 2013;36:287–93.
92. Yu X, Zhao H, Liu L, Cao S, Ren B, Zhang N, et al. A randomized Phase II study of autologous cytokine-induced killer cells in treatment of hepatocellular carcinoma. J Clin Immunol. 2014;34:194–203.
93. Lee JH, Lee JH, Lim YS, Yeon JE, Song TJ, Yu SJ, et al. Adjuvant immunotherapy with autologous cytokine-induced killer cells for hepatocellular carcinoma. Gastroenterology. 2015;148:1383–91.
94. Lesokhin AM, Callahan MK, Postow MA, Wolchok JD. On being less tolerant: enhanced cancer immunosurveillance enabled by targeting checkpoints and agonists of T cell activation. Sci Transl Med. 2015;7:280sr1.
95. Wu Y, Borde M, Heissmeyer V, Feuerer M, Lapan AD, Stroud JC, et al. FOXP3 controls regulatory T cell function through cooperation with NFAT. Cell. 2006;126:375–87.
96. Collins AV, Brodie DW, Gilbert RJ, Iaboni A, Manso-Sancho R, Walse B, et al. The interaction properties of costimulatory molecules revisited. Immunity. 2002;17:201–10.
97. Peggs KS, Quezada SA, Chambers CA, Korman AJ, Allison JP. Blockade of CTLA-4 on both effector and regulatory T cell compartments contributes to the antitumor activity of anti-CTLA-4 antibodies. J Exp Med. 2009;206:1717–25.

98. Bour-Jordan H, Esensten JH, Martinez-Llordella M, Penaranda C, Stumpf M, Bluestone JA. Intrinsic and extrinsic control of peripheral T-cell tolerance by costimulatory molecules of the CD28/B7 family. Immunol Rev. 2011;241:180–205.
99. Sangro B, Gomez-Martin C, de la Mata M, Iñarrairaegui M, Garralda E, Barrera P, et al. A clinical trial of CTLA-4 blockade with tremelimumab in patients with hepatocellular carcinoma and chronic hepatitis C. J Hepatol. 2013;59:81–8.
100. Duffy AG, Ulahannan SV, Makorova-Rusher O, Rahma O, Wedemeyer H, Pratt D, et al. Tremelimumab in combination with ablation in patients with advanced hepatocellular carcinoma. J Hepatol. 2017;66:545–51.
101. Okazaki T, Chikuma S, Iwai Y, Fagarasan S, Honjo T. A rheostat for immune responses: the unique properties of PD-1 and their advantages for clinical application. Nat Immunol. 2013;14:1212–8.
102. Pesce S, Greppi M, Tabellini G, Rampinelli F, Parolini S, Olive D, et al. Identification of a subset of human natural killer cells expressing high levels of programmed death 1: A phenotypic and functional characterization. J Allergy Clin Immunol. 2017;139:335–346.e3.
103. Gao Q, Wang XY, Qiu SJ, Yamato I, Sho M, Nakajima Y, et al. Overexpression of PD-L1 significantly associates with tumor aggressiveness and postoperative recurrence in human hepatocellular carcinoma. Clin Cancer Res. 2009;15:971–9.
104. Zeng Z, Shi F, Zhou L, Zhang MN, Chen Y, Chang XJ, et al. Upregulation of circulating PD-L1/PD-1 is associated with poor post-cryoablation prognosis in patients with HBV-related hepatocellular carcinoma. PLoS One. 2011;6:e23621.
105. El-Khoueiry AB, Melero I, Crocenzi TS, Welling TH, Cheung Yau T, Yeo W, et al. Phase I/II safety and antitumor activity of nivolumab in patients with advanced hepatocellular carcinoma (HCC): CA209-040. J Clin Oncol. 2015;33(18_suppl):LBA101.
106. Segal NH, Antonia SJ, Brahmer JR, Maio M, Blake-Haskins A, Li X, et al. Preliminary data from a multi-arm expansion study of MEDI4736, an anti-PD-L1 antibody. J Clin Oncol. 2014;32:S3002.
107. Abou-Alfa GK, Puig O, Daniele B, Kudo M, Merle P, Park JW, et al. Randomized phase II placebo controlled study of codrituzumab in previously treated patients with advanced hepatocellular carcinoma. J Hepatol. 2016;65:289–95.
108. Konstantinidis KV, Alici E, Aints A, Christensson B, Ljunggren HG, Dilber MS. Targeting IL-2 to the endoplasmic reticulum confines autocrine growth stimulation to NK-92 cells. Exp Hematol. 2005;33:159–64.
109. Imamura M, Shook D, Kamiya T, Shimasaki N, Chai SM, Coustan-Smith E, et al. Autonomous growth and increased cytotoxicity of natural killer cells expressing membrane-bound interleukin-15. Blood. 2014;124:1081–8.
110. Yang B, Liu H, Shi W, Wang Z, Sun S, Zhang G, et al. Blocking transforming growth factor-β signaling pathway augments antitumor effect of adoptive NK-92 cell therapy. Int Immunopharmacol. 2013;17:198–204.
111. Boissel L, Betancur-Boissel M, Lu W, Krause DS, Van Etten RA, Wels WS, et al. Retargeting NK-92 cells by means of CD19- and CD20-specific chimeric antigen receptors compares favorably with antibody-dependent cellular cytotoxicity. Oncoimmunology. 2013;2:e26527.
112. Klingemann H. Are natural killer cells superior CAR drivers? Oncoimmunology. 2014;3:e28147.
113. Lo PH, Urabe Y, Kumar V, Tanikawa C, Koike K, Kato N, et al. Identification of a functional variant in the MICA promoter which regulates MICA expression and increases HCV-related hepatocellular carcinoma risk. PLoS One. 2013;8:e61279.
114. Kohga K, Takehara T, Tatsumi T, Ishida H, Miyagi T, Hosui A, et al. Sorafenib inhibits the shedding of major histocompatibility complex class I-related chain A on hepatocellular carcinoma cells by down-regulating a disintegrin and metalloproteinase 9. Hepatology. 2010;51:1264–73.
115. Krusch M, Salih J, Schlicke M, Baessler T, Kampa KM, Mayer F, et al. The kinase inhibitors sunitinib and sorafenib differentially affect NK cell antitumor reactivity in vitro. J Immunol. 2009;183:8286–94.

116. Yeo W, Chung HC, Chan SL, Wang LZ, Lim R, Picus J, et al. Epigenetic therapy using belinostat for patients with unresectable hepatocellular carcinoma: a multicenter phase I/II study with biomarker and pharmacokinetic analysis of tumors from patients in the Mayo phase II consortium and the cancer therapeutics research group. J Clin Oncol. 2012;30:3361–7.
117. Goto K, Annan DA, Morita T, Li W, Muroyama R, Matsubara Y, et al. Novel chemoimmunotherapeutic strategy for hepatocellular carcinoma based on a genome-wide association study. Sci Rep. 2016;6:38407.
118. Pellom ST Jr, Dudimah DF, Thounaojam MC, Sayers TJ, Shanker A. Modulatory effects of bortezomib on host immune cell functions. Immunotherapy. 2015;7:1011–22.
119. Armeanu S, Krusch M, Baltz KM, Weiss TS, Smirnow I, Steinle A, et al. Direct and natural killer cell-mediated antitumor effects of low-dose bortezomib in hepatocellular carcinoma. Clin Cancer Res. 2008;14:3520–8.

Chapter 3
Antigen-Specific T Cell Responses in Hepatocellular Carcinoma

Eishiro Mizukoshi and Shuichi Kaneko

3.1 Antigenicity and Immunogenicity of HCC

Hepatocellular carcinoma (HCC) arises as a result of (1) chronic hepatitis and liver cirrhosis due to infections with hepatitis B virus (HBV) or hepatitis C virus (HCV), (2) non-alcoholic steatohepatitis, or (3) alcohol-induced cytotoxicity in hepatocytes. Chronic liver inflammation and hepatocyte injury cause genetic and epigenetic changes that lead to formation of cancerous hepatocytes. The changes to the liver can also induce expression of several targets, such as oncofetal antigens and cancer/testis antigens, which are recognized by the host antitumor immune response, possibly leading to the formation of tumors with high antigenicity. In addition, a recent genome-wide association study demonstrated that nonsynonymous somatic mutations occur in solid tumors, including in HCC [1]. Therefore, there is evidence to suggest that HCCs have a relatively high antigenicity.

In addition, it has been reported that tumors in HCC patients contain a large number of lymphocytic infiltrates [2], and that the patients who have undergone surgical removal or liver transplantation show lower risk of recurrence [3]. These data suggest that HCC has high immunogenicity, leading to induction of the antitumor immune response that suppresses tumor progression in HCC patients.

E. Mizukoshi (✉) • S. Kaneko
Department of Gastroenterology, Graduate School of Medicine, Kanazawa University, Kanazawa, Ishikawa 920-8641, Japan
e-mail: eishirom@m-kanazawa.jp

T.F. Greten (ed.), *Immunotherapy of Hepatocellular Carcinoma*,
DOI 10.1007/978-3-319-64958-0_3

3.2 Identification of Tumor-Associated Antigens and Their T Cell Epitopes in HCC

In 1991, Boon and colleagues identified a gene that encodes a melanoma antigen named melanoma-associated antigen (MAGE) [4]. This pioneering study provided the first scientific evidence that the human immune system is capable of clearing tumors in the body by recognizing them as foreign entities. Since then, studies have uncovered the mechanisms of the antitumor immune response involving cytotoxic T lymphocytes (CTLs) that recognize peptides derived from tumor-associated proteins. CTLs recognize the peptides via an interaction between T cell receptors (TCRs) and major histocompatibility complex (MHC) class I molecule complexes that express the peptides on the cell surface.

In the past 10–15 years, several tumor-associated antigens (TAAs) for HCC have been identified, indicating the presence of T cell-mediated immune response in HCC patients (Table 3.1). The following section describes the known TAAs and their CTL epitopes for HCC.

3.2.1 *α-fetoprotein (AFP)*

Since the identification of CTL epitopes for AFP, the underlying immune recognition mechanisms have been studied. AFP is an oncofetal antigen synthesized during fetal development. Although its production is suppressed after birth, it is re-expressed in HCC. As AFP is a self-protein, it was unclear as to whether AFP-specific T cells can be produced and activated to induce an antitumor immune response. However, studies have identified AFP-derived HLA-A2-restricted CTL epitopes in humans, and have shown that CTLs specific to these epitopes can be induced in humans and in HLA-A2 transgenic mice [5]. Several immune-dominant AFP epitopes, including those that are HLA-A24-restricted, have also been identified [6, 7]. These studies demonstrate that the T cell repertoire includes self-antigen-specific CTLs that are not eliminated by central or peripheral tolerance mechanisms. Therefore, self-antigens are one of the attractive targets for immunotherapy against HCC.

3.2.2 *Human Telomerase Reverse Transcriptase (hTERT)*

Human telomerase reverse transcriptase (hTERT) is a catalytic enzyme required for telomere elongation. It is expressed in many cancers, including in HCC. hTERT expression is related to telomerase activity in several cell types including germ, stem and cancer cells, and is associated with the properties of these cells to maintain their cell division. hTERT is also expressed in cancer stem cells that are resistant to

Table 3.1 Tumor associated antigens related HCC and their cytotoxic T lymphocyte epitopes

Antigen	Frequency of expression	T cell epitope	HLA restriction	Year	Author, references
AFP	<80%	$AFP_{137-145}$, $AFP_{158-166}$, $AFP_{325-334}$, $AFP_{542-550}$	A2	2003	Butterfield et al. [5]
		$AFP_{357-415}$, $AFP_{403-411}$	A24	2006	Mizukoshi et al. [6]
NY-ESO-1	<50%	NY-ESO-$1_{157-165}$	A2	2004	Korangy et al. [32]
MAGE-A	<80%	MAGE-$1_{161-169}$	A1	2004	Zerbini et al. [11]
		MAGE-$3_{271-279}$	A2		
		MAGE-$10_{254-262}$	A2	2005	Bricard et al. [10]
SSX-2	<50%	SSX-2_{41-49}	A2	2005	Bricard et al. [10]
hTERT	<80%	$hTERT_{167-175}$, $hTERT_{324-332}$, $hTERT_{461-469}$, $hTERT_{637-645}$, $hTERT_{845-853}$	A24	2006	Mizukoshi et al. [8]
Glypican-3	<70%	$GPC3_{144-152}$	A2	2006	Komori et al. [9]
		$GPC3_{298-306}$	A24		
HCA661	unknown	$HCA661_{110-118}$, $HCA661_{246-254}$	A2	2007	Pang et al. [33]
MRP3	<55%	$MRP3_{503-511}$, $MRP3_{692-700}$, $MRP3_{765-773}$	A24	2008	Mizukoshi et al. [12]
HCA587	<70%	$HCA587_{140-149}$, $HCA587_{144-152}$, $HCA587_{248-256}$	A2	2008	Xing et al. [34]
SART2	100%	$SART2_{93-101}$, $SART2_{161-169}$, $SART2_{899-907}$	A24	2012	Mizukoshi et al. [14]
SART3	100%	$SART3_{109-118}$, $SART3_{315-323}$	A24	2017	Kaji et al. [35]

AFP alpha-fetoprotein, *MAGE* melanoma-associated antigen, *SSX-2* synovial sarcoma/X break-point-2, *hTERT* human telomerase reverse transcriptase, *HCA* hepatocellular carcinoma-associated antigen, *SART* squamous cell carcinoma antigen recognized by T cell

conventional chemotherapy. Therefore, it is an attractive target for cancer immunotherapy. hTERT-derived HLA-A2, A3 and A24-restricted CTL epitopes, and MHC class II-restricted helper T cell epitopes have been identified in many cancers, and measurable amounts of hTERT-specific CTLs have been isolated *ex vivo* from the peripheral blood of HCC patients [8].

3.2.3 Glypican-3 (GPC3)

Glupican-3 (GPC3) is a 65 kDa cell-surface protein consisting of 580 amino acids in the family of heparin sulphate proteoglycans. It was recently identified in a cDNA microarray as an oncofetal antigen expressed specifically in HCC. GPC-derived HLA-A2 and A24-restricted CTL epitopes have been identified, and CTLs that recognize these epitopes have been isolated from the peripheral blood of HCC patients [9].

3.2.4 Synovial Sarcoma X Breakpoint-2 (SSX-2)

Synovial sarcoma X breakpoint-2 (SSX-2) is a cancer/testis antigen overexpressed in HCC. Its CTL epitope was identified in melanoma, and CTLs that recognize the epitope have been isolated from the peripheral blood of HCC patients [10].

3.2.5 Melanoma-Associated Antigen A (MAGE-A)

Antigens in the MAGE-A family, first identified in melanoma, are expressed in many cancers. MAGE-A-derived CTL epitopes have been identified, and CTLs that recognize MAGE-A1 and A3-derived epitopes have been isolated from tumor-infiltrating lymphocytes (TILs) in HCC patients [11]. Studies have also identified CTLs that recognize MAGE-A10-derived epitopes [10].

3.2.6 Multidrug Resistance-Associated Protein 3 (MRP3)

Multidrug resistance-associated protein 3 (MRP3) is an ABC transporter that transports glucuronic acid conjugates as well as a variety of unconjugated organic anion compounds such as antibiotics and anti-inflammatory agents. It is expressed on the basolateral membrane of epithelial cells in the small intestine, where it is believed to be involved in absorption of drugs and bile acid. In liver, it is expressed on the basolateral membrane of hepatocytes along blood vessels, and plays an important role in efflux of unwanted substances from the liver. In addition to normal tissues, its expression has been found in many tumors. MRP3-derived HLA-A2 and A24-restricted CTL epitopes have been identified, and CTLs that recognize the epitopes have been isolated from many cancer patients, including from HCC [12].

In addition to those listed above, there are several TAAs that have been identified in HCC. They include NY-ESO-1, Cyclophyrin-B (Cyp-B), SART, p53, WT-1, β-Catenin and HSP70. CTL epitopes have been identified for some of them, for which the evidence for specific CTL responses have been found in the peripheral blood of HCC patients. Peptides that express some of these CTL epitopes have been used as a vaccine for HCC patients in clinical trials, which will be discussed later.

3.3 Characteristics of Antigen-Specific T Cell Responses in HCC Patients

Identification of HCC-specific T cell epitopes can lead to the development of immunotherapy for HCC. HCC-specific T cell epitopes have also been studied to better understand the mechanisms of immune responses in HCC patients.

3.3.1 Antigen-Specific T Cell Responses in HCC Patients

In general, CTLs that recognize TAA-derived epitopes are obtained by stimulating peripheral blood mononuclear cells (PBMCs) or TILs of patients with candidate peptide epitopes, followed by 1–2 weeks of *in vitro* expansion. Many TAA-derived epitopes have been identified using this method. However, it does not fully recapitulate the T cell frequency and phenotype in patients as it requires long-term *in vitro* culture and stimulation with cytokines such as interleukin-2 (IL-2) or IL-12. This limitation can be overcome by using enzyme-linked immune spot (ELISPOT) or tetramer assays. However, the frequencies of TAA-specific T cells are low in the peripheral blood of cancer patients, including in HCC patients. Thus, there is a certain limit to fully characterize the behavior of TAA-specific T cells in HCC.

A study used the ELISPOT assay to study the frequency of TAA-specific T cells in HCC patients. By comparing a variety of TAA epitopes, the study demonstrated that the frequency of CTLs that are specific to TAA-derived epitopes is 10–60.5 cells/300,000 PMBCs in HCC patients, and that only 3–19% of the patients have CTLs specific to each epitope [13]. These values suggest a weaker host immune response against TAAs compared to that against virus-derived foreign antigens, indicating that there is an insufficient amount of TAA-specific T cells to eliminate tumors.

Studies comparing the immune response against TAA-derived CTL epitopes and the clinical background of HCC patients have generated new information about the host antitumor immune response. For example, it has been reported that different TAAs may elicit different host immune responses. While CTLs against AFP are found more frequently in advanced HCC, those against hTERT, SART and MRP3 can be found in peripheral blood at earlier stages [6, 8, 12, 14].

CTLs specific to some of the TAA epitopes have been obtained by tetramer assay in PMBCs of HCC patients to study their surface markers. For example, hTERT-specific CTLs were found in high frequencies in the peripheral blood of HCC patients who had never been treated with antigen-specific immunotherapy such as peptide vaccines. The memory phenotype of hTERT-specific CTLs varied, with effector being the most frequent, followed by effector memory and central memory [15].

3.3.2 Insufficient Antigen-Specific T Cell Responses

Studies on TAA epitope-specific CTLs by ELISPOT and tetramer assays have identified so-called non-functional CTLs that bind to TAA epitopes but do not produce cytokines such as interferon-γ. Several mechanisms have been proposed to describe the role of non-functional CTLs and the insufficient host antitumor immune response in HCC. Recent studies have also identified a population of immunosuppressive cells, such as regulatory T cells (Tregs) and myeloid-derived suppressor cells (MDSCs), and uncovered the underlying mechanisms of these cells that negatively regulate the antitumor response in HCC. Among different immunosuppressive cells, Tregs have been studied the most to understand the mechanisms of action in suppressing the antitumor immunity. In HCC patients, Tregs are found in PMBCs and TILs, and contribute to tumor progression [16, 17].

MDSC suppresses T cell function by upregulating arginase production that induces Foxp3 and IL-10 expression in $CD4^+$ T cells. Human MDSCs are heterogeneous, and can be divided into granulocytic $CD14^-$ and monocytic $CD14^+$ subtypes. Recent studies have demonstrated that there is an increased number of $CD14^+HLA\text{-}DR^{-/low}$ MDSCs in the peripheral blood of HCC patients [18, 19], and that the number of MDSCs in the peripheral blood after locoregional therapy is negatively correlated with the frequencies of TAA-specific T cells [20]. These studies indicate that the immunosuppressive cells lead to an insufficient TAA-specific immune response.

3.3.3 TAA-Specific T Cell Responses in HCC Treatments

Studies in several cancers have shown that tumors remaining from thermoablation regress spontaneously. This observation suggests that locoregional therapies may induce bystander effects resulting from the TAA-specific T cell response. Indeed, studies on HCCs demonstrated that radiofrequency ablation (RFA) and transarterial chemoembolization (TACE) induce tumor-specific immune responses [21, 22]. For example, an experimental study reported that RFA treatment of a tumor implanted on one side of a mouse led to growth delay in a contralateral tumor, suggesting that the bystander effect involves RFA-induced activation of immune cells such as $CD8^+$ T cells, $CD4^+$ T cells and macrophages [23].

Studies also demonstrated that, in HCC patients who were treated with RFA or TACE, the frequencies of TAA-specific CTLs increase in the peripheral blood after treatment [20, 24]. In this study, however, the treatment-induced antitumor immune response was transient. This suggests that while treatments that induce cellular apoptosis or necrosis trigger antitumor immunity, the resulting antitumor response is insufficient to suppress tumor recurrence after treatment.

Recent studies have further demonstrated that the recurrence rate is significantly lower after RFA when the frequency of TAA-specific CTLs in the peripheral blood is higher after the treatment [20]. This evidence indicates that tumor recurrence may be suppressed when locoregional therapies are followed by immunotherapy in HCC.

3.4 Antitumor Immunity Induced by Antigen-Specific T Cell Therapies in HCC

The first step in establishing the treatment strategies exploiting the antigen-specific T cell immune response is to identify HCC-specific antigens and their T cell epitopes. As HCC is associated with liver dysfunction, immunotherapy should be targeted to tumor cells while sparing healthy hepatocytes for it to be safe and effective. As described earlier, many TAAs and their T cell epitopes for HCC have been identified over the past 10–15 years. Table 3.2 summarizes the clinical trials that made use of peptide vaccines including TAA-derived T cell epitopes.

3.4.1 Antigen-Specific T Cells Induced by Dendritic Cell Therapy

Dendritic cell therapy for HCC involves the use of dendritic cells that are (1) pulsed with TAA-derived peptides, or (2) isolated from patients' PBMCs and infused intratumorally. One such method used dendritic cells that were pulsed with HLA-A2-restricted AFP-derived peptides. While the treatment increased AFP-specific CTLs in 6 out of 10 HCC patients, there were no effects on reducing tumor size [25].

Dendritic cells are activated upon recognition of apoptotic cells. Upon activation, they differentiate into mature dendritic cells to enhance antitumor immunity. In HCC, dendritic cell therapy based on intratumoral infusion is being tested in patients who received treatment with TACE or RFA to investigate whether the therapy induces antigen-specific T cells. Although clinical evidence is limited, some studies demonstrated induction of CTLs that recognize antigen (e.g. AFP, hTERT)-derived epitopes by direct intratumoral infusion of dendritic cells, leading to a decreased recurrence rate after locoregional therapies [26].

Table 3.2 Clinical trials of peptide vaccines for HCC

Setting for peptides, HLA restriction	No. of patients	Responses	Year	Author, references
AFP-derived peptides + Montanide adjuvant, HLA-A2	6	No PR or CR	2003	Butterfield et al. [25]
hTERT-derived peptides + cyclophosphamide + GM-CSF multiple	40	No PR or CR	2010	Greten et al. [27]
GPC3-derived peptides + Montanide adjuvant, HLA-A24 and A2	33	1/33 PR and 19/33 SD	2012	Sawada et al. [28]
SART2-derived peptides + Montanide adjuvant, HLA-A24	12	Immune response	2012	Mizukoshi et al. [14]
hTERT-derived peptides + Montanide adjuvant, HLA-A24	14	Prolonged recurrence-free survival and immune response	2015	Mizukoshi et al. [15]
MRP3-derived peptides + Montanide adjuvant + HAIC, HLA-A24	12	1/12 PR and 9/12 SD	2015	Mizukoshi et al. [36]
SART3-derived peptides + Montanide adjuvant, HLA-A24	12	Immune response	2017	Kaji et al. [35]
AFP-derived peptides + Montanide adjuvant, HLA-A24	20	15 patients were assessed, 1/15 CR and 8/15 SD	2017	Mizukoshi et al. [29]

GM-CSF granulocyte-macrophage colony stimulating factor, *HCC* hepatocellular carcinoma, *AFP* alpha-fetoprotein, *hTERT* human telomerase reverse transcriptase, *GPC3* glypican-3, *SART* squamous cell carcinoma antigen recognized by T cells, *CR* complete response, *PR* partial response, *SD* stable disease

3.4.2 Antigen-Specific T Cells Induced by Peptide Vaccines

Since the discovery of the MAGE gene by Boon and colleagues, immunotherapy trials using tumor antigen-derived peptides have been conducted for many cancer types around the world. Although these clinical studies demonstrated antitumor effects, such as reduction of tumors and suppression of progressive cancer development, complete response (CR) or partial response (PR) has rarely been achieved. Clinical studies suggest that, while the efficacy against advanced cancers may be limited when used alone, peptide vaccines have a significant potential to prevent tumor recurrence, and to prolong survival and time-to-progression. As such, many clinical studies have been conducted to date to test the efficacy of peptide vaccines in several cancers.

Peptide vaccines have been evaluated in clinical trials for HCC. The combination of hTERT-derived peptide vaccines and cyclophosphamide was tested in 40 patients with advanced HCC. The study showed that the immune response was not triggered for the peptide, and that there was no case of CR or PR [27]. On the other hand, a study using HLA-A24-restricted hTERT-derived peptide demonstrated that peptide-specific CTLs were induced in 71.4% of the patients. In this study, the effector memory phenotype was dominant in the induced CTLs [15].

Another study investigated the use of GPC3-derived peptide in 33 patients with advanced HCC. After the treatment, 1 patient achieved PR and 19 patients achieved stable disease (SD) for over 2 months [28]. Of the 19 patients with SD, 4 patients exhibited evidence for tumor necrosis and reduction of tumor size. The results of the study supported the notion of TAA-targeted immunotherapy for HCC.

A study using an HLA-A24-restricted AFP-derived peptide in advanced HCC patients demonstrated that CR and over 2 years of SD can be achieved [29]. This study was performed with patients who did not respond to conventional treatments, such as surgical resection, RFA, TACE, hepatic arterial infusion chemotherapy (HAIC) and sorafenib, demonstrating that the peptide vaccine approach is promising for HCC treatment. Furthermore, the frequencies of peptide-specific T cells increased in the peripheral blood after administration of the vaccine for those patients whose tumors responded to the AFP-derived peptide vaccine. Analysis of the peptide-specific TCRs revealed the presence of TCRs that have a strong binding affinity for AFP-derived CTL epitopes and are cytotoxic to target cells expressing the epitopes. Therefore, the efficacy of peptide vaccines likely depends on the number of TCRs induced by the vaccine as well as the number of TCRs with a high binding affinity to TAA-derived peptides.

3.4.3 Induction of Antigen-Specific TCRs

Adoptive T cell therapy using TILs has demonstrated clinical efficacy in some cancers including melanoma. However, the number of T cells that have tumor-specific TCRs and have antitumor effects is limited, making it challenging to isolate and expand the cell population. Thus, with some exceptions, the use of adoptive T cell therapy has been limited to the treatment of malignant melanoma.

To overcome this limitation, a technique was recently developed to enable manufacturing of a large number of tumor-specific T cells for adoptive T cell transfer. The technique involved transfer of TCR genes from tumor-specific T cells into lymphocytes collected from the peripheral blood of patients. Using this technique, a clinical trial demonstrated that adoptive transfer of MART-1 TCR transgenic T cells leads to reduction of tumor size [30].

Currently, TAA-specific TCRs have been obtained in many cancers. In HCC, TCR genes that recognize AFP, hTERT and GPC3-derived T cell epitopes have been cloned. Furthermore, previously uncharacterized TCRs can now be identified by a novel technique that enables the cloning of single cells. The technique involves a rapid cloning system which enables single-cell isolation of TAA-derived epitope-specific CTLs, cloning of the TCR gene and validation of the TCR specificity to the epitopes in less 10 days [31]. Using this method, AFP-specific TCRs were studied in healthy volunteers and in HCC patients receiving AFP-derived peptide vaccines. The study showed that although AFP-specific T cells existed in the peripheral blood of healthy volunteers, there were only 1–2 TCR repertoires for different epitopes [29]. The number of TCR repertoires increased in patients whose tumors responded to the peptide vaccine. Lymphocytes from the peripheral blood of healthy volunteers were used to manufacture genetically modified T cells that express the AFP-specific TCR gene. The transgenic T cells were highly cytotoxic to target cells expressing the epitope, indicating that the adoptive therapy using AFP TCR transgenic T cells is promising.

In summary, immunotherapy for HCC is anticipated to have significant potential in HCC given that the HCC-specific TAAs have been identified and the antigen-specific T cell responses have been well characterized. Further development of immunotherapy in HCC will depend on the identification of highly immunogenic antigen-derived T cell epitopes, such as neoantigens, as well as a better understanding of the mechanisms underlying antitumor immunity. These studies should lead to the development of novel immunotherapies for HCC that presumably involve the combination of immunotherapeutic approaches engaging multiple mechanisms.

Conflict of Interest The authors disclose no conflicts of interest.

References

1. Vogelstein B, Papadopoulos N, Velculescu VE, Zhou S, Diaz LA Jr, Kinzler KW. Cancer genome landscapes. Science. 2013;339:1546–58.
2. Yoong KF, McNab G, Hubscher SG, Adams DH. Vascular adhesion protein-1 and ICAM-1 support the adhesion of tumor-infiltrating lymphocytes to tumor endothelium in human hepatocellular carcinoma. J Immunol. 1998;160:3978–88.
3. Wada Y, Nakashima O, Kutami R, Yamamoto O, Kojiro M. Clinicopathological study on hepatocellular carcinoma with lymphocytic infiltration. Hepatology. 1998;27:407–14.
4. van der Bruggen P, Traversari C, Chomez P, Lurquin C, De Plaen E, Van den Eynde B, et al. A gene encoding an antigen recognized by cytolytic T lymphocytes on a human melanoma. Science. 1991;254:1643–7.
5. Butterfield LH, Koh A, Meng W, Vollmer CM, Ribas A, Dissette V, et al. Generation of human T-cell responses to an HLA-A2.1-restricted peptide epitope derived from alpha-fetoprotein. Cancer Res. 1999;59:3134–42.
6. Mizukoshi E, Nakamoto Y, Tsuji H, Yamashita T, Kaneko S. Identification of alpha-fetoprotein-derived peptides recognized by cytotoxic T lymphocytes in HLA-A24+ patients with hepatocellular carcinoma. Int J Cancer. 2006;118:1194–204.
7. Thimme R, Neagu M, Boettler T, Neumann-Haefelin C, Kersting N, Geissler M, et al. Comprehensive analysis of the alpha-fetoprotein-specific CD8+ T cell responses in patients with hepatocellular carcinoma. Hepatology. 2008;48:1821–33.
8. Mizukoshi E, Nakamoto Y, Marukawa Y, Arai K, Yamashita T, Tsuji H, et al. Cytotoxic T cell responses to human telomerase reverse transcriptase in patients with hepatocellular carcinoma. Hepatology. 2006;43:1284–94.
9. Komori H, Nakatsura T, Senju S, Yoshitake Y, Motomura Y, Ikuta Y, et al. Identification of HLA-A2- or HLA-A24-restricted CTL epitopes possibly useful for glypican-3-specific immunotherapy of hepatocellular carcinoma. Clin Cancer Res. 2006;12:2689–97.

10. Bricard G, Bouzourene H, Martinet O, Rimoldi D, Halkic N, Gillet M, et al. Naturally acquired MAGE-A10- and SSX-2-specific CD8+ T cell responses in patients with hepatocellular carcinoma. J Immunol. 2005;174:1709–16.
11. Zerbini A, Pilli M, Soliani P, Ziegler S, Pelosi G, Orlandini A, et al. Ex vivo characterization of tumor-derived melanoma antigen encoding gene-specific CD8+cells in patients with hepatocellular carcinoma. J Hepatol. 2004;40:102–9.
12. Mizukoshi E, Honda M, Arai K, Yamashita T, Nakamoto Y, Kaneko S. Expression of multidrug resistance-associated protein 3 and cytotoxic T cell responses in patients with hepatocellular carcinoma. J Hepatol. 2008;49:946–54.
13. Mizukoshi E, Nakamoto Y, Arai K, Yamashita T, Sakai A, Sakai Y, et al. Comparative analysis of various tumor-associated antigen-specific t-cell responses in patients with hepatocellular carcinoma. Hepatology. 2011;53:1206–16.
14. Mizukoshi E, Fushimi K, Arai K, Yamashita T, Honda M, Kaneko S. Expression of chondroitin-glucuronate C5-epimerase and cellular immune responses in patients with hepatocellular carcinoma. Liver Int. 2012;32:1516–26.
15. Mizukoshi E, Nakagawa H, Kitahara M, Yamashita T, Arai K, Sunagozaka H, et al. Immunological features of T cells induced by human telomerase reverse transcriptase-derived peptides in patients with hepatocellular carcinoma. Cancer Lett. 2015;364:98–105.
16. Fu J, Xu D, Liu Z, Shi M, Zhao P, Fu B, et al. Increased regulatory T cells correlate with CD8 T-cell impairment and poor survival in hepatocellular carcinoma patients. Gastroenterology. 2007;132:2328–39.
17. Takata Y, Nakamoto Y, Nakada A, Terashima T, Arihara F, Kitahara M, et al. Frequency of CD45RO+ subset in CD4+CD25(high) regulatory T cells associated with progression of hepatocellular carcinoma. Cancer Lett. 2011;307:165–73.
18. Hoechst B, Ormandy LA, Ballmaier M, Lehner F, Kruger C, Manns MP, et al. A new population of myeloid-derived suppressor cells in hepatocellular carcinoma patients induces CD4(+) CD25(+)Foxp3(+) T cells. Gastroenterology. 2008;135:234–43.
19. Arihara F, Mizukoshi E, Kitahara M, Takata Y, Arai K, Yamashita T, et al. Increase in CD14+HLA-DR −/low myeloid-derived suppressor cells in hepatocellular carcinoma patients and its impact on prognosis. Cancer Immunol Immunother. 2013;62:1421–30.
20. Mizukoshi E, Yamashita T, Arai K, Sunagozaka H, Ueda T, Arihara F, et al. Enhancement of tumor-associated antigen-specific T cell responses by radiofrequency ablation of hepatocellular carcinoma. Hepatology. 2013;57:1448–57.
21. Zerbini A, Pilli M, Penna A, Pelosi G, Schianchi C, Molinari A, et al. Radiofrequency thermal ablation of hepatocellular carcinoma liver nodules can activate and enhance tumor-specific T-cell responses. Cancer Res. 2006;66:1139–46.
22. Ayaru L, Pereira SP, Alisa A, Pathan AA, Williams R, Davidson B, et al. Unmasking of alpha-fetoprotein-specific CD4(+) T cell responses in hepatocellular carcinoma patients undergoing embolization. J Immunol. 2007;178:1914–22.
23. Iida N, Nakamoto Y, Baba T, Nakagawa H, Mizukoshi E, Naito M, et al. Antitumor effect after radiofrequency ablation of murine hepatoma is augmented by an active variant of CC Chemokine ligand 3/macrophage inflammatory protein-1alpha. Cancer Res. 2010;70:6556–65.
24. Mizukoshi E, Nakamoto Y, Arai K, Yamashita T, Mukaida N, Matsushima K, et al. Enhancement of tumor-specific T-cell responses by transcatheter arterial embolization with dendritic cell infusion for hepatocellular carcinoma. Int J Cancer. 2010;126:2164–74.
25. Butterfield LH, Ribas A, Dissette VB, Lee Y, Yang JQ, De la Rocha P, et al. A phase I/II trial testing immunization of hepatocellular carcinoma patients with dendritic cells pulsed with four alpha-fetoprotein peptides. Clin Cancer Res. 2006;12:2817–25.
26. Nakamoto Y, Mizukoshi E, Kitahara M, Arihara F, Sakai Y, Kakinoki K, et al. Prolonged recurrence-free survival following OK432-stimulated dendritic cell transfer into hepatocellular carcinoma during transarterial embolization. Clin Exp Immunol. 2011;163:165–77.

27. Greten TF, Forner A, Korangy F, N'Kontchou G, Barget N, Ayuso C, et al. A phase II open label trial evaluating safety and efficacy of a telomerase peptide vaccination in patients with advanced hepatocellular carcinoma. BMC Cancer. 2010;10:209.
28. Sawada Y, Yoshikawa T, Nobuoka D, Shirakawa H, Kuronuma T, Motomura Y, et al. Phase I trial of a glypican-3-derived peptide vaccine for advanced hepatocellular carcinoma: immunologic evidence and potential for improving overall survival. Clin Cancer Res. 2012;18:3686–96.
29. Mizukoshi E. Association between high-avidity T-cell receptors, induced by alpha fetoprotein-derived peptides, and anti-tumor effects in patients with hepatocellular carcinoma. Gastroenterology. 2017;152:1395–406.
30. Morgan RA, Dudley ME, Wunderlich JR, Hughes MS, Yang JC, Sherry RM, et al. Cancer regression in patients after transfer of genetically engineered lymphocytes. Science. 2006;314:126–9.
31. Kobayashi E, Mizukoshi E, Kishi H, Ozawa T, Hamana H, Nagai T, et al. A new cloning and expression system yields and validates TCRs from blood lymphocytes of patients with cancer within 10 days. Nat Med. 2013;19:1542–6.
32. Korangy F, Ormandy LA, Bleck JS, Klempnauer J, Wilkens L, Manns MP, et al. Spontaneous tumor-specific humoral and cellular immune responses to NY-ESO-1 in hepatocellular carcinoma. Clin Cancer Res. 2004;10:4332–41.
33. Pang PH, Chan KT, Tse LY, Chan RC, Cheung YK, Sin FW, et al. Induction of cytotoxic T cell response against HCA661 positive cancer cells through activation with novel HLA-A *0201 restricted epitopes. Cancer Lett. 2007;256:178–85.
34. Xing Q, Pang XW, Peng JR, Yin YH, Li Y, Yu X, et al. Identification of new cytotoxic T-lymphocyte epitopes from cancer testis antigen HCA587. Biochem Biophys Res Commun. 2008;372:331–5.
35. Kaji K, Mizukoshi E, Yamashita T, Arai K, Sunagozaka H, Fushimi K, et al. Cellular Immune Responses for Squamous Cell Carcinoma Antigen Recognized by T Cells 3 in Patients with Hepatocellular Carcinoma. PLoS One. 2017;12:e0170291.
36. Mizukoshi E, Nakagawa H, Kitahara M, Yamashita T, Arai K, Sunagozaka H, et al. Phase I trial of multidrug resistance-associated protein 3-derived peptide in patients with hepatocellular carcinoma. Cancer Lett. 2015;369:242–9.

Chapter 4
Immune Checkpoint Inhibitors for the Treatment of Hepatocellular Carcinoma

Mercedes Iñarrairaegui, Delia D'Avola, and Bruno Sangro

4.1 Immune Checkpoint Molecules and the Immune Response Against Tumors

The adaptive immune response against cancer is a complex process that takes place at different sites. Following capture of cell debris, dendritic cells (DC) uptake and process tumor associated antigens (TAA) inside the tumor, become activated and migrate to the regional lymph nodes, where they present the TAA inside a major histocompatibility complex (MHC) class II molecule to CD4+ T cells [1]. Antigen recognition then stimulates CD4+ T cells to proliferate and produce interferon gamma (IFN-γ) in a process called type 1 T helper cell (Th1) polarization. Th1 polarization occurs in the presence of type I interferon and interleukin 12 (IL-12) released by DC, and is governed by intracellular co-stimulatory signals resulting from CD28 on the CD4+ T cell membrane binding to CD80 and CD86 on the DC surface. Th1 cells license DCs for cross-presentation of TAA to CD8+ T cells, thus assisting in the development of CD8+ cytotoxic T lymphocytes (CTL). Circulating CTL eventually migrate to tumor sites, where they can interact with their cognate MHC class I-TAA complex on the membrane of the tumor cells. The antitumor activity of TAA-specific CD8+ T cells relies on their ability to produce IFN-γ, which inhibits tumor cell growth, and on their cytotoxic activity mediated by the release of granzyme B and perforin, and by the interaction with FAS and TRAIL receptors on tumor cells [2]. In HCC, the relevant role of the Th1 response is supported by clinical findings showing that the expression of Th1 cytokines (IL-1α, IL-1β, IL-2 and IFN-γ) in tumor tissue is associated with good prognosis, whereas

M. Iñarrairaegui • D. D'Avola • B. Sangro (✉)
LiverUnit, Clínica Universidad de Navarra-IDISNA, Pamplona, Spain

Centro de Investigación Biomédica en Red de Enfermedades Hepáticas y Digestivas (CIBEREHD), Pamplona, Spain
e-mail: minarra@unav.es; ddavola@unav.es; bsangro@unav.es

T.F. Greten (ed.), *Immunotherapy of Hepatocellular Carcinoma*,
DOI 10.1007/978-3-319-64958-0_4

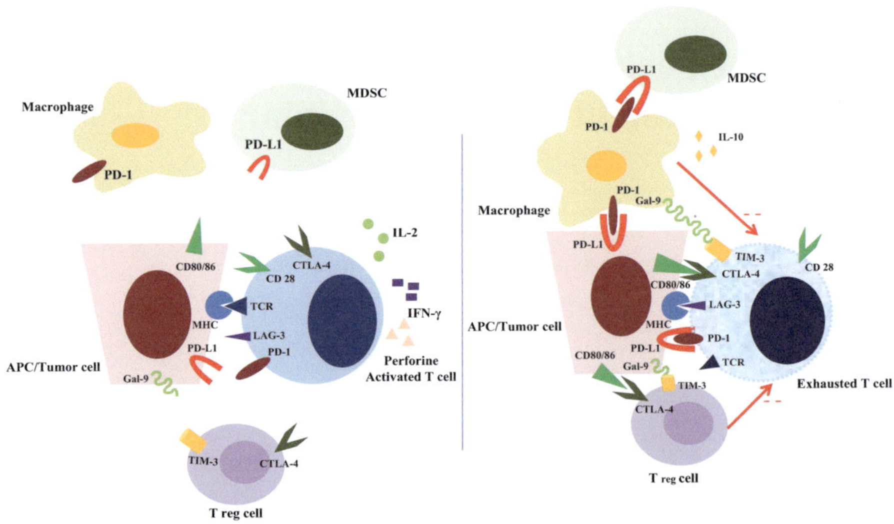

Fig. 4.1 Interplay of the main immune check points in liver cancer. CTLA-4 binds CD80 and CD86, antagonizing the interaction of CD28 with these receptors. PD-1 binds PD-L1 and inhibits CD4+ and CD8+ activation (Tcell exhaustion). LAG-3 synergizes the inhibitory effect of PD-1 on T cell function by binding MHC class I molecules. TIM-3 binds different ligands and inhibits T cell activation and enhances Treg activity

Effect of the main immune check points in liver cancer: CTLA-4 is able to bind CD80 and CD86, antagonizing the interaction of CD28 with these receptors, that results into a decreased T cell activation upon APC antigen presentation. PD-1 expressed on T-cells and other immune cells such as macrophages bind PD-L1 expressed on APC, tumor cells and MDSC and inhibits both CD8+ activation and proliferation and CD4+ activation by blocking the TCR signaling, decreasing the secretion of IFN-gamma from T cells (T-cell exhaustion). On tumor associated macrophages, the binding of PD-1 to its ligand leads to an increased secretion of IL-10 that exert inhibitory effect on T-cells. LAG-3 synergizes inhibitory effect of PD-1 on T cell function by binding MHC class I molecules. TIM-3 expressed on T-cells and T-reg cells and tumor associated macrophages. It binds different ligands such as Gal-9 expressed on APC, Tumor cells and macrophpages. The main effect of TIM-3 is the inhibition of T-lymphocytes activation and the enhancement of T-reg cells activity

Th2 cytokines (IL-4, IL-5 and IL-10) are upregulated in advanced HCC with vascular invasion and metastasis [3].

Immune checkpoints are a specific subtype of membrane-bound molecules that provide fine-tuning of the immune response. A comprehensive review of their variety and functions can be obtained in [4, 5] and their key functions are summarized in Fig. 4.1. Immune checkpoints are expressed in different cell types involved in the immune response, including B and T cells, natural killer (NK) cells, DC, tumor associated macrophages (TAM), monocytes, and myeloid-derived suppressor cells (MDSC). Under physiological conditions, most of these molecules display an immunosuppressive activity that prevents T cell overactivation during the immune response against infection and limits collateral tissue damage. The immune checkpoints most studied in human cancer are cytotoxic T-lymphocyte protein 4 (CTLA-4), programmed cell death protein 1 (PD-1), lymphocyte activation gene 3 protein (LAG-3), B and T lymphocyte attenuator (BTLA), and T-cell immunoglobulin and mucin-domain containing (TIM-3).

CTLA-4 is essential for the activation of CD4+ T cells and the priming phase of the immune response. Expressed on activated T cells, CTLA-4 has great affinity for CD80 and CD86 and may thus antagonize the interaction of CD28 with these receptors, with resulting decreased T cell activation upon antigen presentation. CTLA-4 is also constitutively expressed on regulatory T cells (Treg). Treg are CD4+ T cells that can be characterized by the presence of CD25, CTLA-4, CD62L and FoxP3 molecules in their membrane. Activated by TCR engagement concurrent with IL-10 and TGF-β signaling, Treg inhibit the immune response through various mechanisms including depletion of IL-2 and secretion of immunosuppressive factors such as TGF-β, IL-10 or adenosine, as well as competition with co-stimulatory CD28 via CTLA-4. Hence, CTL-4 is also required for Treg to exert its suppressive activity on activated Tcells [6]. But the role of CTLA-4 is not restricted to the priming phase. Inside the tumor, CTLA-4 also promotes immunosuppression by inducing Treg activity and differentiation and upregulating IDO and IL-10 in DC [7].

PD-1 is a key factor in the effector phase of the immune response. It is expressed by activated CD8+ and CD4+ T cells, B cells, NK, Treg, MDSC, monocytes and DC. PD-L1 and PD-L2 are the ligands of PD-1. PD-1 is expressed in hematopoietic cells, including APC and MDSC, and in different types of parenchymal cells too, while PD-L2 expression is limited to the haematopoietic compartment. PD-L1 is upregulated by various cytokines, particularly IFN-γ. Upon binding to its ligands, PD-1 inhibits CD8+ T cell activation by blocking the TCR signaling, and inhibits CD4+ activation and proliferation through increased secretion of IL-10. Cancer cells may also express PD-L1 and PD-L2 and use this mechanism to escape from immunosurveillance. Indeed, in a situation of chronic antigen exposure such as the tumor microenvironment, IFN-γ produced by TAA-specific T cells induces PD-1 expression on reactive T lymphocytes and upregulates PD-L1 in APC and tumor cells. PD-1–PD-L1 engagement then blocks TCR signaling and inhibits T cell proliferation and secretion of cytotoxic mediators, in a process called T cell exhaustion [8]. The expression of PD-L1 is enhanced by IFN-γ release under the hypoxic conditions present in most tumors.

TIM-3 is a transmembrane protein expressed on cells of the innate and adaptive immune system that interacts with several ligands including phosphatidylserine on the membrane of apoptotic cells, galectin-9 and others. Galectin-9 is a soluble protein produced by cells from many different tissue types (including the liver) that regulates cell differentiation, adhesion and cell death. Evidence indicates that galectin-9 suppresses T-cell responses, which supports the concept that TIM-3 acts as an inhibitory receptor for T cells. Furthermore, CD8+ Tim-3+ T cells in animal models coexpress PD-1, and these dual-expressing cells exhibit greater defects in both cell-cycle progression and effector cytokine production IL-2, TNF, and IFN-γ than cells that express PD-1 alone. The TIM-3 pathway may thus cooperate with the PD-1 pathway to promote the development of a severe dysfunctional phenotype in CD8+ T cells in cancer [9].

LAG-3 is a membrane protein that binds MHC class II molecules with high affinity, thus reducing the co-stimulatory functions of DC. LAG-3 is not expressed on resting T cells but is upregulated upon activation. It is a marker of exhausted T cells and acts synergistically with PD-1 to promote cancer evasion from immunity [10, 11]. Finally, BTLA is an immunoglobulin-like molecule expressed by several immune cells including B and T lymphocytes, NK and antigen presenting cells. BTLA is able to inhibit T cell proliferation and cytokine production upon binding to its ligand, herpesvirus entry mediator (HVEM), which can be expressed in HCC [12, 13].

4.2 The Relevance of Immune Checkpoint Molecules in the Immunological Background of Liver Cancer

The liver has a unique immunological milieu compared to any other organ of the human body. The interaction between different resident cells, such as Kupffer cells (KC), hepatic stellate cells (HSC), liver sinusoidal endothelial cells (LSEC), and different types of immune cells, such as DC, NK, T or B lymphocytes, contribute to maintain a predominantly immunotolerant microenvironment in the liver. This is probably a protective mechanism aimed to limit the inflammatory response that may result from the continuous exposure of the liver parenchyma to different types of antigens transported from the gut through the portal circulation. Indeed, activation of the cellular immune response inside the liver parenchyma is limited by different mechanisms. Particularly by a high expression of inhibitory membrane molecules such as PD-1 and PDL-1, a low expression of costimulatory molecules such as CD80 and CD86, and a high concentration of immunosuppressive cytokines such as IL-10. While this immunotolerant environment can be considered a protective mechanism under physiological conditions, it may have detrimental consequences when liver cancer arises.

The immune response is relevant to HCC development and behavior, and the detection of a specific immune response against HCC has been associated with less advanced tumors and better prognosis [14]. As a matter of fact, different studies have shown that among HCC patients treated by liver resection or transplantation, a dense lymphocytic infiltration of the tumor carries a better prognosis [15, 16]. The configuration of such infiltrate is also important. Tumor infiltrating Treg correlate with poor outcome in HCC patients after resection [17] while an inverse correlation has been shown between the number of MDSC and patient outcome after RFA ablation [18]. On the other hand, most HCC tumors develop in the setting of cirrhosis due to chronic viral infection. Chronic IFN-γ release resulting from chronic inflammation may also lead to Tcell exhaustion. Increasing evidence suggests that the exhaustion of the immune response may impair the prognosis of HCC. The inability of the tumor-infiltrating CD8+ lymphocytes to produce IFN-γ upon antigen stimulation has been described in human HCC [14]. High expression of PD-1 and PD-L1 in liver cancer tissue has been reported to predict poor prognosis in HCC patients undergoing liver resection with an increased rate of recurrence after resection; and is associated to more aggressive tumor characteristics [19, 20].

But PD-1/PD-L1 is not the only pathway that has been involved in HCC. An overexpression of LAG-3 in tumor infiltrating CD8+ lymphocytes compared to peripheral lymphocytes was observed in patients with HCC related to HBV infection [21]. In patients with HBV-related HCC, an overexpression of TIM-3 on tumor infiltrating CD4+ and CD8+ T lymphocytes has been reported and found to be associated to replicative senescence of T cells [22]. In an animal homograft model of liver cancer, TIM-3 expression in TAM enhanced tumor growth in vivo [23]. The high concentration of TGF-b produced by liver tumor cells seems to upregulate TIM-3 in TAM and induces an M2 phenotype in these cells. Moreover, TIM-3 is able to promote the alternative activation of TAM in a TGF-beta independent mechanism [23]. The high levels of cytokines, mainly IL-6 and IL-10, produced by M2 TAM may ultimately promote tumor growth. In patients with HCC, the expression of TIM-3 in monocytes and TAM strongly correlated with higher tumor grades and poor survival [23].

As mentioned above, BTLA is able to inhibit T cell proliferation and cytokine production upon binding to its ligand, herpesvirus entry mediator (HVEM), which can be expressed in HCC [12, 13]. A high expression of HVEM expression in HCC is associated with reduced lymphocyte infiltration, diminished levels of effector T cell mediators, and worse prognosis after resection [24]. It has recently been shown that in patients with HCC the majority of BTLA+ CD4+ T cells also express PD-1 [25]. This suggests that BTLA may identify a highly dysfunctional CD4+ T cells population within liver cancer. Interestingly, a high concentration of BTLA+ PD1+ CD4+ T cells, but not of BTLA- PD1+ CD4 T cells, was associated with more advanced HCC stages.

4.3 Clinical Experience with the Use of Checkpoint Inhibitors in Hepatocellular Carcinoma

All these preclinical information provides a valid rationale for an immunologic approach to the treatment of HCC based on the interaction with immune checkpoints. Clinical studies have only recently been conducted but the results are more than encouraging. There is no hyperbole in saying that checkpoint inhibitors have revolutionized cancer care. Signals delivered by immune checkpoints plays a major role in the induction and maintenance of tumor immune tolerance. Monoclonal antibodies that block negative signals for T lymphocytes may allow the amplification of the T cell response, avoidance of T cell exhaustion, or elimination of Treg. These compounds have shown a wide spectrum of anticancer activity that resulted in a survival advantage over standard therapies in several cancer types, including melanoma, head and neck squamous carcinoma, non-small cell lung cancer, bladder cancer, renal cell cancer, or Hodgkin's lymphoma [26–31].

In the field of HCC, clinical development has focused on CTLA-4 and PD-1/PD-L1 pathways (Tables 4.1 and 4.2).Tremelimumab is a fully human IgG2

Table 4.1 Trial design and patient characteristics in reported clinical trials using immune checkpoint inhibitors in HCC

Author, year	Study phase	Agent	Dose	Target	N	Etiology	BCLC B/C	Child A	Prior sorafenib
Sangro, 2013 [33]	2	Tremelimumab	15 mg/kg every 90 days	CTLA-4	21 17[a]	HCV	28/57%	57%	24%
Duffy, 2016 [35]	1b/2	Tremelimumab + RFA/TACE	3.5 to 10 mg/kg every4 weeks × 6 doses and then every 3 months	CTLA-4 + tumor ablation[b]	32 19[a]	No infected, HBV and HCV	25/75%	86%	65%
El-Khoueiry A, 2017 [38]	1b/2	Nivolumab	0.1 to 10 mg/kg every 2 weeks (3 mg/kg on expansion phase)	PD-1	262[c]	No infected, HBV and HCV	12/88%	98.4%	69%

[a]Number of patients evaluable for tumor response
[b]5 weeks after 1st dose
[c]48 patients from dose-escalation phase and 214 from dose-expansion phase

Table 4.2 Results reported in prospective clinical trials using immune checkpoint inhibitors in HCC

	Efficacy				Safety Any grade (grade ≥ 3) CTCAE			
Author, Year	ORR	SD	TTP (95% CI), months	OS (95% CI), months	Rash	Pruritus	Diarrhea	ASAT
Sangro, 2013 [33]	17.6%	58.8%	6.48 (3.95–9.14)	8.2 (4.64–21.34)	65% (5%)		30% (5%)	70% (45%)
Duffy, 2016 [35]	26%	63%	7.7 (4.7–19.4)	12.3 (9.3–15.4)	15% (0)	9.3% (0)	6.2% (0)	34% (22%)
El-Khoueiry, 2017 [38]	18%	44%	nr	15 m[a] (9.6–20.2 m)	16.7% (0.7%)	20% (0.3%)	12% (1.1%)	10% (5%)

[a]Dose-escalation phase. Not reported in those-expansion phase

monoclonal antibody that blocks the binding of cytotoxic T-lymphocyte-associated antigen 4 (CTLA-4). As explained, CTLA-4 at the immune synapse outcompetes the binding of the CD28 co-stimulatory receptor to CD80 and CD86 with much superior avidity. This binding sends an inhibitory signal that serves as a natural brake for T cell activation. Tremelimumab blocks the inhibitory effect of CTLA-4, and therefore enhances T cell activation and proliferation [32]. Among CTLA-4 targeted therapies, tremelimumab was the first molecule to be clinically evaluated in HCC. Our group led a phase II, non-controlled, multicenter trial that targeted the population of patients with HCC and chronic HCV infection who were not eligible for surgery or locoregional therapy [33]. We had the dual intention to test the antitumor and antiviral activity of tremelimumab in a single study. The study was 80% powered to reject the null hypothesis that objective response rate did not exceed 5% at a 0.05 level of significance if true objective response rate was >25%. Based on a Simon's optimal 2-stage design 3 tumor responses among 17 evaluable patients were needed to reject the null hypothesis. Twenty-one patients with fairly advanced disease (57% were at BCLC C stage) were enrolled, most of them (57%) having progressed to previous therapies. Importantly, a significant proportion of patients (42.9%) were in Child-Pugh stage B, indicating some degree of liver dysfunction. Patients received what we now know is a suboptimal dose of 15 mg/kg tremelimumab every 90 days to a maximum of 4 doses unless tumor progression or unacceptable toxicities occurred. Despite this suboptimal dosing, 3 partial responses were observed among 17 evaluable patients and the trial was found to be positive based on the initial assumptions. Stable disease was the best response in 10 additional patients, accounting for a remarkable disease control rate of 76.4%. Quite importantly, almost half (45%) of these stabilizations lasted longer than 6 months. Among 11 patients that had alpha-fetoprotein levels higher than 100 ng/ml at baseline, 36% showed a > 50% drop following treatment, providing further evidence of antitumor activity. Median time to progression was 6.48 months (CI 95% 3.95–9.14 months). Although potentially biased by a long tumor assessment interval, this prolonged time to progression compares favorably with several targeted agents as shown in Table 4.3. The observed overall survival of 8.2 months (CI 95% 4.64–21.34 months)

Table 4.3 Systemic agents for the second line treatment of advanced HCC: a perspective to understand the data from immune-oncology agents

			Patient profile				Overall survival (months)		Time to progression (months)	
Trial	Agent	n	Child B	ECOG >0	EHD	MVI	Median	95%CI	Median	95%CI
Randomized trials with targeted agents										
BRISK-PS	Brivanib	263	7%	43%	65%	31%	9.4	nr	4.2	nr
	Placebo	132	9%	39%	64%	18%	8.2	nr	2.7	nr
Tivantinb 2 L	Tivantinib	71	4%	42%	69%	60%	6.6	4–6-9.0	1.6	1.4–2.8
	Placebo	36	3%	42%	78%	64%	6.2	3.8–9-4	1.4	1.4–1.5
EVOLVE-1	Everolimus	362	2%	40%	74%	32%	7.6	6.7–8.4	3.0	2.8–4.0
	Placebo	184	1%	43%	73%	33%	7.4	6.3–8.7	2.6	1.5–2.8
REACH-1	Ramucirumab	283	2%	44%	73%	29%	9.2	8.1–10.6	3.5	2.8–4.5
	Placebo	282	2%	46%	71%	28%	7.6	6.0–9.3	2.6	1.6–2.8
RESORCE	Regorafenib	379	1%	35%	70%	29%	10.6	9.1–12.1	3.2	2.9–4.2
	Placebo	194	3%	33%	76%	28%	7.8	6.3–8.8	1.5	1.4–1.6
Single arm trials with immune checkpoint inhibitors										
	Tremelimumab	21	43	28%	9%	28%	8.2	4.6–21.3	6.5	3.9–9.1
	Tremelimumab + ablation	32	14	75%	45%	nr	12.3	9.3–15.4	7.7	4.7–19.4
CheckMate040	Nivolumab	262	2%	nr	76%	8%	15.0	9.6–20.2	nr	nr

Refs.: BRISK-PS [52], Tivantinib 2L [53], EVOLVE [54], REACH-1 [55], RESORCE [56], Tremelimumab [33, 35], CheckMate-040 [38]

was not much different from what could be observed in patients receiving placebo in second-line trials but the high proportion of Child B patients in this cohort likely had a significant impact in this outcome.

A significant antiviral effect was also observed, with a decrease in median viral load from 3.78×10^5 IU/ml at day 0 to 3.02×10^4 IU/ml at day 120 ($n = 11, p = 0.011$), and 1.69×10^3 IU/ml at day 210 ($n = 6$, $p = 0.017$). The progressive course of this decline in viral load was observed in most patients followed for at least 3 months, and three patients had a transient complete viral response during follow-up. The immunological origin of this viral response was supported by the fact that it was observed in 75% of patients with an immune response (defined as a >5-fold increase at any time in the sum of IFN-g-producing cells against viral antigen) versus 20% of patients with no immune response. Patients with an early decrease in IL-6 had a higher chance of having a viral response (100%) than those with increased values at that time (43%).The antitumoral effect was not associated to this antiviral effect or to patient characteristics including systemic inflammatory signals such as C reactive protein. The lack of repeated tumor biopsies precludes any interpretation of the mechanism behind the antitumor activity while the expansion in circulating Treg following tremelimumab therapy was in line with observations in other tumor types [34].

Regarding safety, tremelimumab was well tolerated, with few patients experiencing grade 3 disabling adverse events, even in the presence of liver dysfunction among patients in the Child-Pugh B class. No patient received systemic steroids and there were no treatment-related deaths. An itching skin rash was the most frequent adverse event (65%), which was successfully managed with topic agents and oral antihistamine drugs. Diarrhea was observed in 30% of patients but reached grade 3 in only one patient. A remarkable rise in serum transaminases was observed after the first dose in more than half of the patients, being grade 3 or higher in 45% of cases but with no other signs of liver dysfunction. This effect on transaminases was transient, did not recur in the following cycles, and was not related to the antitumor or antiviral responses, or with changes in circulating cytokines.

Following the same path, a second trial tested a very appealing hypothesis i.e. whether an antigenic stimulation provided by means of incomplete tumor ablation using percutaneous radiofrequency (RFA) or transarterial chemoembolization (TACE) could safely enhance the effects of tremelimumab [35]. The rationale for this combination is based on the fact that RFA or TACE could induce immunogenic tumor cell death and this in turn could stimulate a peripheral systemic immune response that may be further amplified by immune checkpoint blockade. In a phase I/II trial increasing doses of tremelimumab were given followed by subtotal tumor ablation and tumor response was evaluated in those lesions not targeted by RFA, cryoablation or TACE procedures. This was a pilot study with no specific sample size assumptions. Thirty-two patients with mostly advanced HCC (75% at BCLC C stage) were enrolled, 78% having progressed to previous therapies. Patient characteristics were therefore quite similar to the previous study except that liver function was preserved in the vast majority of patients, with only 14% of patients in Child-Pugh class B. Most patients (75%) had viral hepatitis as cause of liver cirrhosis.

Enrolled patients were treated this time with an optimal dose of tremelimumab at two dose levels (3.5 and 10 mg/kg IV) given every 4 weeks for a total of 6 doses, followed by 3-monthly infusions until off-treatment criteria were met. The interventional radiologic procedure (TACE for BCLC B and thermal ablation for BCLC C patients) was performed 5 weeks after first dose of tremelimumab. Nineteen patients were evaluable for response because they had measurable lesions that were not targeted by RFA or TACE. Of these patients, partial response was recorded in 5 patients (26%), and stable disease in 12 patients (63%), accounting for a disease control rate of 89%. Again, almost half (45%) of the stabilizations lasted longer than 6 months and median time to progression was 7.4 months (95% CI 4.7–9.4 months). Given the small number of patients in both tremelimumab trials, the small differences in response rates and time to progression seem of little relevance but provide a signal of the consistency of the antitumor effect. The better overall survival of 12.3 months (95% CI 9.3–15.4 months) in the combination trial could be explained on the basis of the good liver function but a true enhancing effect of prior ablation may not be ruled out.

Regarding safety, one relevant observation was that there was no clear trend in adverse events across the different dose cohorts. The most common clinical toxicity was pruritus, although less frequent than in the previous trial (9%), and was predominantly grade 1. Less frequent side effects were diarrhea (6%), autoimmune pneumonitis (3%) and angioedema (3%). Again, the most frequent laboratory alteration was hypertransaminasemia, which occurred in 34% of patients and was grade 3 or 4 in 21% of them. The antiviral activity was also confirmed in this trial. The HCV viral load of 14 quantifiable patients decreased after 3 months in 12 patients, with a median HCV viral load decrease from 1275×10^3 UI/ml to 351×10^3 UI/ml.

This trial was enriched with important correlative studies. The amount of peripheral blood CD3, CD4, CD8, CD38 and HLA-DR positive cells was analyzed after every cycle by multicolor flow cytometry. Tumor biopsies were obtained from some patients immediately before ablation (after 2 doses of tremelimumab). The number of cytotoxic T cells (CD3 and CD8 positive) was measured by immunohistochemistry in these samples and compared to archival samples obtained prior to enrollment. Interestingly, the number of peripheral activated CD4+ and CD8+ T cells increased after tremelimumab. Such increase was especially intense and sustained for CD8 + T cells. Immune cell tumor infiltration was observed in all 12 patients in whom post-tremelimumab tumor samples could be evaluated. Among those 6 patients with paired tumor samples, an increase in both CD3+ and CD8+ cells was observed although the differences were not statistically significant, likely because of the small number of cases. Patients with objective remissions in non-ablated lesions had a higher post-tremelimumab CD3+ and CD8+ infiltration compared to non-responders. Unfortunately the effect of ablation on T-cell infiltration could not be evaluated and in the absence of a remarkable difference in patient outcomes, the synergy between TACE/RFA and CTLA-4 blockade remains an appealing hypothesis to be confirmed.

The encouraging signs of antitumor activity of tremelimumab in advanced HCC and its good safety profile in cirrhotic patients of viral etiology, provided a strong reason to test other checkpoints inhibitors [36]. The PD-L1/PD-1 pathway provides another mechanism of tumor-induced immune tolerance. PD-1 expression on effector phase CD8 + T cells is increased in HCC patients compared to cirrhotic patients or healthy controls [19]. And indeed, HCC patients with higher numbers of tumor infiltrating and circulating PD-1 + CD8+ T cells showed earlier and more frequent disease progression after hepatic resection. PD-L1 is also highly expressed on peritumoral stromal cells (Kupffer cells, LSEC, and monocytes) as well as cancer cells, promoting a PD-L1/PD-1 pathway-driven inhibition of antitumor T cell responses [20, 37]. Thus, a strong rationale supports the use of PD-1 and PD-L1 blocking antibodies against HCC. Building on the experience with tremelimumab, we helped develop the first clinical trial to assess the safety and clinical benefit of nivolumab, a fully human IgG4 monoclonal antibody targeting PD-1,as a first or second-line treatment in patients with advanced HCC across different etiologies (HCV infection, HBV infection, non-viral cirrhosis) [38].

The target population of the CheckMate 040 trial included patients with intermediate or advanced HCC and preserved liver function (Child-Pugh A) that were candidates to systemic therapy and had progressed or were intolerant to sorafenib or had refused this drug. First, a dose-escalation cohort of 48 patients received doses that ranged from 0.3 mg/kg to 10 mg/kg every 2 weeks with the primary endpoint of establishing the safety and tolerability of nivolumab in HCC patients. Afterwards, the 3 mg/kg dose level was chosen for an expansion cohort of 214 patients in whom the primary endpoint was efficacy evaluated as objective response rate using RECIST 1.1 criteria. Patients in this expansion cohort were divided in four specific groups of uninfected patients progressing to sorafenib, uninfected patients naïve or intolerant to sorafenib, patients with HCV infection and patients with HBV infection. In both cohorts, HBV-infected patients had to be on effective antiviral therapy (circulating viral DNA < 100 UI/ml) [38].

Contrary to the tremelimumab trials, this study recruited patients from Europe, Asia and America. Most were at the advanced BCLC stage C (88%), had extrahepatic metastases (68%), and had received prior systemic therapy (76%), mainly sorafenib. Treatment was by and large well tolerated. Adverse events were observed at similar rates across dose levels and a maximal tolerated dose was not reached. The most frequent symptomatic adverse events in the large expansion cohort treated with 3 mg/kg were rash (23%), pruritus (21%) and diarrhea (13%), that were usually mild. Grade 3 or higher treatment-related symptomatic adverse events occurred in less than 2% of patients. Hypertransaminasemia was the most frequent laboratory alteration (20%) reached grade 3 or higher in only 5% of patients. Regarding etiologies, rates of symptomatic treatment-related AEs were comparable in the uninfected and HCV- or HBV-infected cohorts. Overall, frequencies of grade 3/4 treatment-related AEs and treatment-related serious AEs overall were 20% and 7%, respectively, while no treatment-related deaths occurred. Immune related hepatitis needing steroid therapy occurred very rarely. Only 3% of patients discontinued nivolumab due to treatment-related adverse events and no treatment-related deaths were reported.

Convincing signs of efficacy were reported. In the escalation and expansion cohorts, objective tumor responses were reported in 15% and 20% of patients, respectively. And they were meaningful, durable responses that lasted for a median of 17 months. An additional 45% of patients had stable disease that was frequently durable too, lasting more than 6 months in most cases. The majority of objective responses occurred during the first 3 months of treatment. It has to be stressed that response rates were similar across different etiologies, and both in sorafenib-naive and sorafenib-exposed patients. This signs of efficacy were consistent with the 9-month survival rate of 70% reported in the large expansion cohort and the median overall survival of 15 months (95% CI 9.6–20.2 months) reported in the dose-escalation cohort with a longer follow-up. This median survival was observed irrespective of prior sorafenib treatment, and compares well with any other phase 2 or 3 clinical trial of targeted agents including regorafenib, the first agent shown to prolong survival following sorafenib in a selected group of sorafenib-tolerant patients. Indeed, these results support nivolumab as a viable second-line therapy following sorafenib (Table 4.3).

A comprehensive biomarker analysis has not yet been reported for this trial. Expression of PD-L1 prior to nivolumab was studied in fresh or archival tumor specimens. The rate was remarkably low. Even with a cut-off for positivity of 1% of tumor cells exhibiting membrane PD-L1 staining of any intensity, only 20% of 174 evaluable patients had PD-L1 positive tumors. Objective remissions were observed in 26% of PD-L1 positive patients and 19% of PD-L1 negative patients. The more relevant rate of PD-L1 expression in tumor stromal cells and its association with response to nivolumab have not been reported yet.

4.4 Ongoing Studies and Potential Combinations

Building upon this experience, clinical development around immune checkpoints in HCC has thriven. A summary of ongoing studies is provided in Table 4.2. Some of them are designed to help define the place of specific agents in the treatment paradigm for HCC. This group includes two pivotal phase 3 trials comparing nivolumab vs. sorafenib as first-line systemic therapy for advanced HCC, and pembrolizumab vs. best supportive care as second-line therapy for patients that progress or are intolerant to sorafenib. Some others are designed to expand the potential of immunotherapy based on the interaction with checkpoint molecules in several ways. The potential rationale according to treatment platforms is illustrated in Fig. 4.2.

The activity of PD-1/PD-L1 inhibition not only in HCC but also across tumor types makes it a sound backbone for combinatorial strategies. The simultaneous blockade of different checkpoints may produce synergistic effects and has shown impressive results in patients with melanoma [39]. Dual blockade of PD-L1 and the non-redundant CTLA-4 is attempted in a phase 1b cohort of the Checkmate 040 where different doses of ipilimumab (a CTLA-4 blocking IgG1 monoclonal antibody) and nivolumab are tested [38]. Another trial with a 1b/2 design is testing the

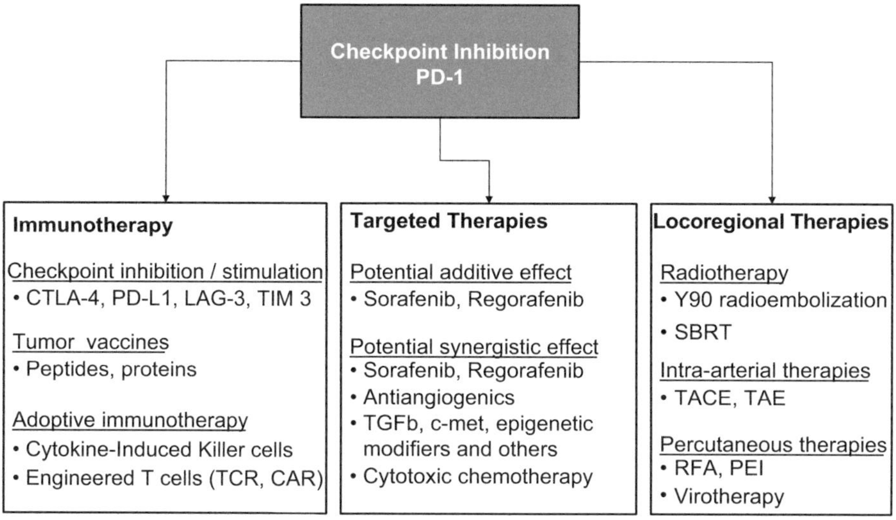

Fig. 4.2 Potential combinations for therapeutic development in immunotherapy of HCC (*TCR* T cell receptor, *CAR* chimeric antigen receptor, *TACE* transarterial chemoembolization, *TAE* transarterial (bland) embolization, *RFA* radiofrequency ablation, *PEI* percutaneous ethanol injection)

combination of durvalumab (a PD-L1 blocking monoclonal antibody) and tremelimumab compared to each agent as monotherapy. Durvalumab has shown a good safety profile in a small cohort of HCC patients treated in a basket trial [40].

Stimulation of co-stimulatory molecules such as CD137 (4-1BB), CD134 (OX40), glucocorticoid-induced tumor necrosis factor receptor (GITR) or CD40 may potentiate the effector functions activated T cells and NK, constrain the suppressive activity of Treg, and enhance antibody-dependant cellular cytotoxicity. Combining PD-1/PD-L1 inhibition with stimulation of these co-stimulatory molecules would simultaneously release the brakes and press the gas pedal of the immune response. As a matter of fact, this strategy has proven effective in HCC models [41] and deserves clinical testing.

Inhibition of oncogenic pathways may have an effect on the antitumor immune response. For instance, BRAF inhibition in melanoma may increase the expression of melanoma differentiation antigens and HLA molecules on tumor cells, induction of PD-1 expression, and inhibition of suppressive cytokines as IL-10 [42]. Even more importantly, BRAF inhibition may increase CD8+ T cell tumor infiltration, a potential hallmark for immuno-oncology agents effectiveness. Regarding antiangiogenic drugs, VEGF modulates antitumor immunity through different mechanisms including the expansion of suppressive cell subtypes such as Treg and MDSC, inhibition of DC maturation, or suppression of T cell responses [43]. Again in melanoma patients, combination of ipilimumab and the VEGFR antagonist bevacizumab produced intense tumor infiltration by CD8+ T cells and dendritic macrophages as well as high numbers of peripheral memory T cells [44]. Little is known about the specific immune effect of sorafenib. Studies performed in animal HCC models showed that sorafenib-induced hypoxia may inhibit the immune response by increasing intratumoral expression of PD-L1 and enhancing the recruitment of Treg and M2 macrophages [45]. In this study the combination of an anti-PD1 antibody and sorafenib was not more effective than sorafenib alone. A different study suggested that sorafenib increases the local recruitment of tumor-associated neutrophils and ultimately populates the tumor stroma with macrophages and Treg, thus promoting an immunosuppressive environment [46]. In this study, depletion of tumor-associated neutrophils combined with sorafenib led to a stronger anti-tumoral activity compared to sorafenib alone. In the clinical setting, the combination of sorafenib and PD-1 blockade will be tested.

The release or expression of tumor antigens and the immune-adjuvant like effect of tumor irradiation is the basis for the well-known phenomenon of the abscopal effect [47, 48]. In a sense, radiotherapy may act as a "local tumor vaccine". In animal models, a variety of synergistic effects occur when radiation therapy is combined with CTLA-4 blockade including diversification of the TCR repertoire of tumor infiltrating lymphocytes and modeling of the repertoire of expanded T cell clones [49]. The potential synergy of this combination has been also suggested in advanced melanoma patients [50]. In HCC, selective internal radiation therapy or radioembolization is increasingly used as a locoregional therapy for different stages. Clinical trials trying to exploit this potential synergy are underway (Table 4.4). The ability of other forms of locoregional treatment of HCC such as TACE or RFA to

Table 4.4 Ongoing clinical trials testing immuno-oncology agents in HCC

Phase	Population	Agents	Target	NCT number
IO agents as monotherapy				
1b/2	1L and 2L	Nivolumab	PD-1	01658878
2	2L	Pembrolizumab	PD-1	02702414
3	1L	Nivolumab vs. Sorafenib	PD-1	02576509
3	2L	Pembrolizumab vs. best supportive care	PD-1	02702401
IO agents in combination with other IO agents				
1b/2	2L	Nivolumab + Ipilimumab	PD-1 & CTLA-4	01658878
1b/2	1L and 2L	Tremelimumab + Durvalumab vs. Durvalumab vs. Tremelimumab	PD-L1 & CTLA-4	02519348
IO agents in combination with non-IO agents				
1b/2		PDR001 vs PDR001 + Capmatinib	PD-1 & c-met	02795429
1b/2		Nivolumab + CC-122	PD-1 & pleiotropic pathway modifier	02859324
1b/2		Nivolumab + Galunisertib	PD-1 &TGFb	02423343
1a/b		Durvalumab + Ramucirumab	CTLA4 & VEGFR2	02572687
1b		Pembrolizumab + Nintendanib	PD-1 &multikinase	02856425
1		Pembrolizumab + Lenvatinib	PD-1 &multikinase	03006926
1b		PDR001 + Sorafenib	PD-1 &multikinase	02988440
1b/2		Nivolumab + Y90 radioembolization	PD-1 & radiation	03033446 02837029

favor immune responses is much less established. Nevertheless, ongoing clinical trials are taking advantage of the information about the combination of subtotal TACE/RFA cited above. Intratumoral injection of the vaccinia oncolytic virus Pexavec was able to produce distant responses but failed to prove effective in prolonging survival of patients with advanced HCC [51].

Natural interaction between tumor and host defines the amount and specificity of pre-existent tumor reactive T cells. If the number of T cell clones primed by tumor-associated antigens is low (as it could be particularly for tumors with a low mutational load), the tumor immune infiltrate may not be intense enough to benefit from the immune stimulation of checkpoint inhibitors and the efficacy of checkpoint inhibitors would be reduced or abolished. Effective tumor vaccines may overcome this problem. Co-administration of tumor-associated neoantigens and a strong immune adjuvant is the basis of the HEPAVAC project and clinical trial (http://www.hepavac.eu/).

Conflicts of Interest Bruno Sangro has received consulting and/or lecture fees from Adaptimmune, Astra Zeneca, Bayer Healthcare, Bristol-Myers-Squibb, and Medimmune.

Funding Delia D'Avola is the recipient of the Grant for Study Expansion from the Spanish Association for the Study of the Liver (Asociación Espanola para el Estudio del Hígado AEEH) and Cancer Research Grant from Nuovo Soldati Foundation. This work was supported by EC FP7 Project Cancer Vaccine development for Hepatocellular Carcinoma – HEPAVAC (Grant Nr. 602,893), EC H2020 Project Immunology and Immunotherapy of cancer: strengthening the translational aspect – HepaMUT (Grant Nr. AC16/00165), and project PI16/01845, integrated in Plan Estatal de I + D + I 2013–2016 and co-financed by ISCIII-Subdirección General de Evaluación y Fomento de la investigación and Fondo Europeo de Desarrollo Regional (FEDER).

References

1. Anguille S, Smits EL, Bryant C, Van Acker HH, Goossens H, Lion E, et al. Dendritic cells as pharmacological tools for cancer immunotherapy. Pharmacol Rev. 2015;67:731–53.
2. Mittal D, Gubin MM, Schreiber RD, Smyth MJ. New insights into cancer immunoediting and its three component phases-elimination, equilibrium and escape. Curr Opin Immunol. 2014;27:16–25.
3. Budhu A, Forgues M, Ye QH, Jia HL, He P, Zanetti KA, et al. Prediction of venous metastases, recurrence, and prognosis in hepatocellular carcinoma based on a unique immune response signature of the liver microenvironment. Cancer Cell. 2006;10:99–111.
4. Prieto J, Melero I, Sangro B. Immunological landscape and immunotherapy of hepatocellular carcinoma. Nat Rev Hepatol. 2015;12:681–700.
5. Le Mercier I, Lines JL, Noelle RJ. Beyond CTLA-4 and PD-1, the generation Z of negative checkpoint regulators. Front Immunol. 2015;6:418.
6. Wing K, Onishi Y, Prieto-Martin P, Yamaguchi T, Miyara M, Fehervari Z, et al. CTLA-4 control over Foxp3+ regulatory T cell function. Science. 2008;322:271–5.
7. Han Y, Chen Z, Yang Y, Jiang Z, Gu Y, Liu Y, et al. Human CD14+CTLA-4+ regulatory dendritic cells suppress T-cell response by cytotoxic T-lymphocyte antigen-4-dependent IL-10 and indoleamine-2,3-dioxygenase production in hepatocellular carcinoma. Hepatology. 2014;59:567–79.
8. Barber DL, Wherry EJ, Masopust D, Zhu B, Allison JP, Sharpe AH, et al. Restoring function in exhausted CD8 T cells during chronic viral infection. Nature. 2006;439:682–7.

9. Anderson AC. Tim-3: an emerging target in the cancer immunotherapy landscape. Cancer Immunol Res. 2014;2:393–8.
10. Nguyen LT, Ohashi PS. Clinical blockade of PD1 and LAG3 – potential mechanisms of action. Nat Rev Immunol [Internet]. 2015;15:45–56.
11. Triebel F, Jitsukawa S, Baixeras E, Roman-Roman S, Genevee C, Viegas-Pequignot E, et al. LAG-3, a novel lymphocyte activation gene closely related to CD4. J Exp Med. 1990;171:1393–405.
12. Sedy JR, Gavrieli M, Potter KG, Hurchla MA, Lindsley RC, Hildner K, et al. B and T lymphocyte attenuator regulates T cell activation through interaction with herpesvirus entry mediator. Nat Immunol. 2005;6:90–8.
13. Watanabe N, Gavrieli M, Sedy JR, Yang J, Fallarino F, Loftin SK, et al. BTLA is a lymphocyte inhibitory receptor with similarities to CTLA-4 and PD-1. Nat Immunol. 2003;4:670–9.
14. Flecken T, Schmidt N, Hild S, Gostick E, Drognitz O, Zeiser R, et al. Immunodominance and functional alterations of tumor-associated antigen-specific CD8+ T-cell responses in hepatocellular carcinoma. Hepatology. 2014;59:1415–26.
15. Unitt E, Marshall A, Gelson W, Rushbrook SM, Davies S, Vowler SL, et al. Tumour lymphocytic infiltrate and recurrence of hepatocellular carcinoma following liver transplantation. J Hepatol. 2006;45:246–53.
16. Wada Y, Nakashima O, Kutami R, Yamamoto O, Kojiro M. Clinicopathological study on hepatocellular carcinoma with lymphocytic infiltration. Hepatology. 1998;27:407–14.
17. Gao Q, Qiu S-J, Fan J, Zhou J, Wang X-Y, Xiao Y-S, et al. Intratumoral balance of regulatory and cytotoxic T cells is associated with prognosis of hepatocellular carcinoma after resection. J Clin Oncol. 2007;25:2586–93.
18. Arihara F, Mizukoshi E, Kitahara M, Takata Y, Arai K, Yamashita T, et al. Increase in CD14+HLA-DR −/low myeloid-derived suppressor cells in hepatocellular carcinoma patients and its impact on prognosis. Cancer Immunol Immunother. 2013;62:1421–30.
19. Shi F, Shi M, Zeng Z, Qi RZ, Liu ZW, Zhang JY, et al. PD-1 and PD-L1 upregulation promotes CD8(+) T-cell apoptosis and postoperative recurrence in hepatocellular carcinoma patients. Int J cancer. 2011;128:887–96.
20. Gao Q, Wang XY, Qiu SJ, Yamato I, Sho M, Nakajima Y, et al. Overexpression of PD-L1 significantly associates with tumor aggressiveness and postoperative recurrence in human hepatocellular carcinoma. Clin Cancer Res. 2009;15:971–9.
21. Li FJ, Zhang Y, Jin GX, Yao L, Wu DQ. Expression of LAG-3 is coincident with the impaired effector function of HBV-specific CD8+ T cell in HCC patients. Immunol Lett. 2013;150:116–22.
22. Li H, Wu K, Tao K, Chen L, Zheng Q, Lu X, et al. Tim-3/galectin-9 signaling pathway mediates T-cell dysfunction and predicts poor prognosis in patients with hepatitis B virus-associated hepatocellular carcinoma. Hepatology. 2012;56:1342–51.
23. Yan W, Liu X, Ma H, Zhang H, Song X, Gao L, et al. Tim-3 fosters HCC development by enhancing TGF-β-mediated alternative activation of macrophages. Gut. 2015;1–12.
24. Hokuto D, Sho M, Yamato I, Yasuda S, Obara S, Nomi T, et al. Clinical impact of herpesvirus entry mediator expression in human hepatocellular carcinoma. Eur J Cancer. 2015;51:157–65.
25. Zhao Q, Huang Z-L, He M, Gao Z, Kuang D-M. BTLA identifies dysfunctional PD-1-expressing CD4+ T cells in human hepatocellular carcinoma. Oncoimmunology. 2016;5
26. Garon EB, Rizvi NA, Hui R, Leighl N, Balmanoukian AS, Eder JP, et al. Pembrolizumab for the treatment of non-small-cell lung cancer. N Engl J Med. 2015;372:2018–28.
27. George S, Motzer RJ, Hammers HJ, Redman BG, Kuzel TM, Tykodi SS, et al. Safety and efficacy of nivolumab in patients with metastatic renal cell carcinoma treated beyond progression: a subgroup analysis of a randomized clinical trial. JAMA Oncol. 2016;2:1179–86.
28. Ansell SM, Lesokhin AM, Borrello I, Halwani A, Scott EC, Gutierrez M, et al. PD-1 blockade with nivolumab in relapsed or refractory Hodgkin's lymphoma. N Engl J Med. 2015;372:311–9.

29. Petrylak DP, Powles T, Bellmunt J, Braiteh FS, Loriot Y, Zambrano C, et al. A phase Ia study of MPDL3280A (anti-PDL1): updated response and survival data in urothelial bladder cancer (UBC). J Clin Oncol. 2015;Suppl 33: Abstr 4501.
30. Postow MA, Callahan MK, Wolchok JD. Immune checkpoint blockade in cancer therapy. J Clin Oncol. 2015;33:1974–82.
31. Chow LQ, Haddad R, Gupta S, Mahipal A, Mehra R, Tahara M, et al. Antitumor activity of pembrolizumab in biomarker-unselected patients with recurrent and/or metastatic head and neck squamous cell carcinoma: results from the phase Ib KEYNOTE-012 expansion cohort. J Clin Oncol. 2016;34:3838–45.
32. Peggs KS, Quezada SA, Chambers CA, Korman AJ, Allison JP. Blockade of CTLA-4 on both effector and regulatory T cell compartments contributes to the antitumor activity of anti-CTLA-4 antibodies. J Exp Med. 2009;206:1717–25.
33. Sangro B, Gomez-Martin C, de la Mata M, Inarrairaegui M, Garralda E, Barrera P, et al. A clinical trial of CTLA-4 blockade with tremelimumab in patients with hepatocellular carcinoma and chronic hepatitis C. J Hepatol. 2013;59:81–8.
34. Kavanagh B, O'Brien S, Lee D, Hou Y, Weinberg V, Rini B, et al. CTLA4 blockade expands FoxP3+ regulatory and activated effector CD4 + T cells in a dose-dependent fashion. Blood. 2008;112:1175–83.
35. Duffy AG, Ulahannan SV, Makorova-Rusher O, Wedemeyer H, Pratt D, Davis JL, et al. Tremelimumab in combination with ablation in patients with advanced hepatocellular carcinoma. J Hepatol. 2017;66:545–51.
36. Sprinzl MF, Galle PR. Current progress in immunotherapy of hepatocellular carcinoma. J Hepatol [Internet]. 2017;66:482–4.
37. Wang B-J, Bao J-J, Wang J-Z, Wang Y, Jiang M, Xing M-Y, et al. Immunostaining of PD-1/PD-Ls in liver tissues of patients with hepatitis and hepatocellular carcinoma. World J Gastroenterol. 2011;17:3322–9.
38. El-Khoueiry A, Sangro B, Yau T, Crocenzi T, Kudo M, Hsu C, et al. Nivolumab in patients with advanced hepatocellular carcinoma (CheckMate 040): an open-label, non-comparative, phase 1/2 dose escalation and expansion trial. Lancet. 2017;389(10088):2492–502.
39. Larkin J, Chiarion-Sileni V, Gonzalez R, Grob JJ, Cowey CL, Lao CD, et al. Combined nivolumab and ipilimumab or monotherapy in untreated melanoma. N Engl J Med. 2015;373:23–34.
40. Segal HN, Scott A, Brahmer JR, Maio M, Blake-Haskins A, Li X, et al. Preliminary data from a multi-arm expansion study of MEDI4736, an anti-PD-L1 antibody. J Clin Oncol. 2014;32:5s abstr 3002.
41. Morales-Kastresana A, Sanmamed MF, Rodriguez I, Palazon A, Martinez-Forero I, Labiano S, et al. Combined immunostimulatory monoclonal antibodies extend survival in an aggressive transgenic hepatocellular carcinoma mouse model. Clin Cancer Res. 2013;19:6151–62.
42. Hu-Lieskovan S, Robert L, Moreno BH, Ribas A. Combining targeted therapy with immunotherapy in BRAF-mutant melanoma: promise and challenges. J Clin Oncol. 2014;32:2248–54.
43. Kandalaft LE, Motz GT, Busch J, Coukos G. Angiogenesis and the tumor vasculature as antitumor immune modulators: the role of vascular endothelial growth factor and endothelin. Curr Top Microbiol Immunol. 2011;344:129–48.
44. Hodi FS, Lawrence D, Lezcano C, Wu X, Zhou J, Sasada T, et al. Bevacizumab plus ipilimumab in patients with metastatic melanoma. Cancer Immunol Res. 2014;2:632–42.
45. Chen Y, Ramjiawan RR, Reiberger T, Ng MR, Hato T, Huang Y, et al. CXCR4 inhibition in tumor microenvironment facilitates anti-programmed death receptor-1 immunotherapy in sorafenib-treated hepatocellular carcinoma in mice. Hepatology. 2015;61:1591–602.
46. Zhou SL, Zhou ZJ, Hu ZQ, Huang XW, Wang Z, Chen EB, et al. Tumor-associated neutrophils recruit macrophages and T-regulatory cells to promote progression of hepatocellular carcinoma and resistance to sorafenib. Gastroenterology. 2016;150:1646–1658.e17.
47. Mole RH. Whole body irradiation; radiobiology or medicine? Br J Radiol. 1953;26:234–41.

48. Demaria S, Ng B, Devitt ML, Babb JS, Kawashima N, Liebes L, et al. Ionizing radiation inhibition of distant untreated tumors (abscopal effect) is immune mediated. Int J Radiat Oncol Biol Phys. 2004;58:862–70.
49. Victor CT-S, Rech AJ, Maity A, Rengan R, Pauken KE, Stelekati E, et al. Radiation and dual checkpoint blockade activate non-redundant immune mechanisms in cancer. Nature. 2015;520:373–7.
50. Postow MA, Callahan MK, Barker CA, Yamada Y, Yuan J, Kitano S, et al. Immunologic correlates of the abscopal effect in a patient with melanoma. N Engl J Med. 2012;366:925–31.
51. Heo J, Reid T, Ruo L, Breitbach CJ, Rose S, Bloomston M, et al. Randomized dose-finding clinical trial of oncolytic immunotherapeutic vaccinia JX-594 in liver cancer. Nat Med. 2013;19:329–36.
52. Llovet JM, Decaens T, Raoul JL, Boucher E, Kudo M, Chang C, et al. Brivanib in patients with advanced hepatocellular carcinoma who were intolerant to sorafenib or for whom sorafenib failed: results from the randomized phase III BRISK-PS study. J Clin Oncol. 2013;31:3509–16.
53. Santoro A, Simonelli M, Rodriguez-Lope C, Zucali P, Camacho LH, Granito A, et al. Tivantinib for second-line treatment of advanced hepatocellular carcinoma: a randomised, placebo-controlled phase 2 study. Lancet Oncol. 2013;14:55–63.
54. Zhu AX, Kudo M, Assenat E, Cattan S, Kang YK, Lim HY, et al. Effect of everolimus on survival in advanced hepatocellular carcinoma after failure of sorafenib: the EVOLVE-1 randomized clinical trial. JAMA. 2014;312:57–67.
55. Zhu AX, Park JO, Ryoo BY, Yen CJ, Poon R, Pastorelli D, et al. Ramucirumab versus placebo as second-line treatment in patients with advanced hepatocellular carcinoma following first-line therapy with sorafenib (REACH): a randomised, double-blind, multicentre, phase 3 trial. Lancet Oncol. 2015;16:859–70.
56. Bruix J, Qin S, Merle P, Granito A, Huang YH, Bodoky G, et al. Regorafenib for patients with hepatocellular carcinoma who progressed on sorafenib treatment (RESORCE): a randomised, double-blind, placebo-controlled, phase 3 trial. Lancet. 2017;389:56–66.

Chapter 5
Cytokine-Induced Killer Cells for the Adjuvant Treatment of Patients with HCC

Jeong-Hoon Lee and Jung-Hwan Yoon

5.1 Need for Adjuvant Therapy in HCC

Most cases of hepatocellular carcinoma (HCC) occur in patients with well-known risk factors such as chronic hepatitis B virus (HBV) or hepatitis C virus (HCV), and nonalcoholic steatohepatitis, as well as other risk factors such as chronic alcoholism and liver cirrhosis. Thus, a regular surveillance program for populations with such risk factors may allow the diagnosis of HCC at early stage, which is candidate for potentially curative treatment. In fact, in Japan and Taiwan, >50% of HCC cases were diagnosed at either a very early or early stage owing to the implementation of a nationwide regular surveillance program [1]. However, the long-term prognosis of HCC is still poor even after curative treatment because of high risk of recurrence in the remnant liver.

In most other malignancies, adjuvant therapy is usually indicated for patients who undergo surgical treatment for locally advanced tumors, but not at a very early or early stage. For example, adjuvant systemic chemotherapy is indicated for gastric cancer of stages I_B or II_A, colon cancer of stages II or III, and non-small cell lung cancer of stages II or III_A but not for any cancer of stage I or I_A since there is a low risk of tumor recurrence after curative treatment. However, in contrast, the National Cancer Institute recommends enrolling very early or early stage HCC patients for clinical trials of adjuvant therapy [2]. A very high risk of tumor recurrence, even after potentially curative treatment, is the basis of this exclusive recommendation for early HCC. Potentially curative treatment for early HCC and gastric cancer resulted in 5-year recurrence-free survival rates of <30% [3] and greater than 90%, respectively [4]. This difference may be linked to a significant difference in 5-year survival rates: 76% in early HCC and >90% in early gastric cancer.

J.-H. Lee • J.-H. Yoon (✉)
Department of Internal Medicine and Liver Research Institute,
Seoul National University College of Medicine, Seoul, South Korea
e-mail: yoonjh@snu.ac.kr

T.F. Greten (ed.), *Immunotherapy of Hepatocellular Carcinoma*,
DOI 10.1007/978-3-319-64958-0_5

The recurrence of HCC can be classified according to its timing. Early recurrence refers to recurrence within 2 years after tumor treatment and usually occurs by the metastasis of remnant tumor cells. Late recurrence means recurrence after 2 years and is thought to be a *de novo* recurrence from diseased liver [5]. Consequently, early recurrence is closely related to tumor factors including safety margin, vessel invasion, multiple tumor nodules, and serum levels of α-fetoprotein. In contrast, fibrosis and inflammation determined by a HBV and HCV load and histological inflammatory activity is associated with late recurrence.

Numerous efforts have been made to reduce recurrence in the form of the development of novel adjuvant therapies; however, the benefit of such remains uncertain. Till now, the only proven therapy that reduces the risk of HCC recurrence is antiviral treatment for HBV-related HCC patients. However, all adjuvant therapy which aimed to kill residual tumor cells failed to show efficacy. For example, polyprenoic acid (an acyclic retinoid) and sorafenib (a multikinase inhibitor) failed to decrease tumor recurrence in phase III trials. Therefore, current international guidelines do not recommend adjuvant therapy after curative treatment [6, 7]. In response, to overcome the lack of an effective adjuvant therapy, many scientists are trying to utilize adoptive immunotherapy.

5.2 Mechanisms of Immune Tolerability of HCC

Cellular immunity, in particular, T cell-mediated cytotoxicity, is the main armory of the human immune system deployed to combat cancers. Cytotoxic T cells may recognize tumor cells by interactions between the T cell receptor and an antigenic-peptide present on the type I major histocompatibility complex (MHC). Using perforin, T cells induce the formation of pores in the tumor cell membrane, via which granzyme enters to induce tumor cell apoptosis. Malignant cells develop multiple immune evasion mechanisms to avoid host immunity (Fig. 5.1). For example, they may hide themselves by reducing the production of tumor antigens and class I MHC molecules on their surface. Another immune evasion technique demonstrated by tumor cells is their disruption of T cell signaling, leading to the induction of T cell apoptosis in response to their expression of interleukin (IL)-10, transforming growth factor-β (TGF-β), and receptor-binding cancer antigen expressed on SiSo cells 1 (RCAS1). As well as T cells, tumor cells also act to suppress the immune response by the induction of myeloid-derived suppressor cells (MDSC) and regulatory T cells (T_{reg}s). In addition, X-linked inhibitor of apoptosis (XIAP) and FADD-like IL-1β-converting enzyme-inhibitory protein (c-FLIP) interfere with apoptosis induction by T cells, surviving [8].

In HCC, an environment suitable for immune evasion occurs due to: (i) the inherent tolerogenic nature of liver, (ii) hepatitis virus-related immunosuppression, and (iii) immune impairment induced by the tumor itself.

The liver is known as "an immune-privileged organ" that shows an inherent tolerogenicity in both healthy and diseased states. The liver continuously contacts

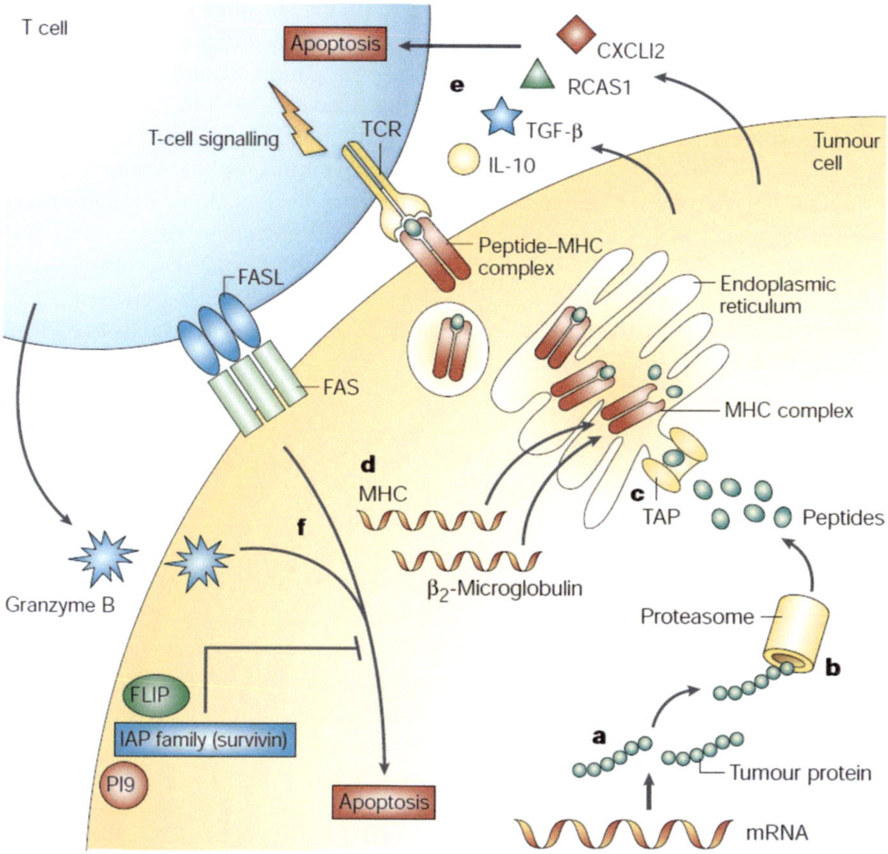

Fig. 5.1 Mechanisms of immune evasion. Tumors may use several means of escaping the effects of the immune system: (**a**) cytokines and other molecules expressed by tumor cells may induce T-cell apoptosis or inhibit T-cell signaling; (**b**) tumor surface MHC molecules, which present tumor peptide epitopes to T-cell receptors (TCR), may not be expressed correctly; (**c**) the transporter that moves peptides to the endoplasmic reticulum for the formation of peptide-MHC complexes may malfunction; (**d**) the proteasome may change its methods of breaking down tumor protein into peptides for antigen presentation; and (**e**) tumor antigen expression becomes decreased or is absent. In the face of apoptosis induced by T cells, the expression of immunoprotective agents (the IAP family, FLIP, and PI9) is upregulated by tumor cells to thwart the activity of granzyme B and interactions by FAS-FAS ligands
CXCL12 chemokine (C-X-C motif) ligand 12, *FLIP* FLICE (FADD-like interleukin-1β–converting enzyme)–like inhibitory protein, *IAP* inhibitor of apoptosis protein, *IL-10* interleukin-10, *PI9* proteinase inhibitor 9, *RCAS1* receptor-binding cancer antigen expressed on SiSo cells, *TGF-β* transforming growth factor-β (Reprinted by permission from Macmillan Publishers Ltd.: (NATURE REVIEWS CANCER) [8], copyright (2002))

and clears toxins delivered via the portal circulation. In other to avoid aberrant immunity, the liver has developed a redundant immune regulation mechanism. Hepatocytes prime naïve T cells without co-stimulation, resulting in defective effector function [9]. Immune tolerance in the liver is related to the presence of antigen presenting cells (APCs; i.e. liver sinusoidal endothelial, hepatic dendritic [DCs], and Kupffer cells). Kupffer cells (liver-resident macrophages) produce anti-inflammatory factors, including TGF-β, IL-10, and prostaglandin E2, and reduce antigen-specific $CD8^+$ T cells [10, 11]. Myeloid DC precursors differentiate into IL-10–secreting DCs in the liver. When IL-10–secreting hepatic DCs prime naïve $CD4^+$ T cells, T_{reg}s are induced and the antigen recall process is impaired. More importantly, the expression of programmed death-ligand 1 (PD-L1) on liver sinusoidal endothelial cells and its interaction with programmed death (PD)-1 on T cells leads to the induction of antigen-specific T cell tolerance [10].

Immunosuppression is also enhanced by the most common underlying etiologies of HCC, chronic hepatitis B and C. In response to both virus-specific and unrelated antigens, T cell proliferation and the production of IL-2 are inhibited in a chronic HBV infection and T_{reg}s accumulate in the liver. And with regard to infection with chronic hepatitis C, a reduced effector function of natural killer (NK) cells leads to the inhibition of the maturation of DC in response to various maturation signals. The expression of inhibitory immune checkpoints, such as PD-1, on T cells is enhanced, resulting in dysfunction of both HCV-specific and -nonspecific T cells.

HCC itself also displays a series of immune evasion mechanisms similar to other malignancies. In patients with HCC, the quantity and quality of myeloid DC and NK cells are decreased. Aberrantly activated monocytes in HCC express abundant PD-1 and impair anti-tumor T cell immunity. Immune suppressor cells, including MDSCs and T_{reg}s, accumulate in HCC patients and correlate with tumor volume.

Such mechanisms of immune tolerability of HCC may need to be overcome to develop an effective immunotherapy option.

5.3 Adoptive Immunotherapies for HCC

Chronic inflammation is closely linked to the development and progression of HCC. For example, IL-6, and tumor necrosis factor-α (TNF-α) were found to promote the development of HCC as described by previous studies [12]. After the establishment of HCC cells, mutual interactions between tumor and immune cells, which can exist during chronic inflammation, may create favorable conditions for tumor cell survival [13]. Tumor-associated macrophages, T_{reg}s, and MDSCs may act as immune suppressors and facilitate tumor immune evasion [14]. Tumor growth factor-β, IL-10, and IL-17 are important cytokines that also display an immune suppression function. In contrast to immune suppressors, the numbers and effectiveness of effector cells, such as NK, dendritic, and cytotoxic T cells, are downregulated within the tumor microenvironment [15]. Furthermore, mutations increase during the growth of tumors allowing these to avoid the immune system [16]. Antigen presenting cells and $CD8^+$ T cell activities are also impaired, which leads to the attenuation of their cytotoxic effects dependent on MHC classes [17]. A proportion of HCC cells also express low levels of MHC molecules. Such major constraints of the cytotoxic immune response against HCC can be circumvented by likely beneficial approaches such as increasing and decreasing, respectively, the numbers of MHC-unrestricted direct cytotoxic effector and immune suppressor cells.

5.3.1 *Tumor-Infiltrating Lymphocytes*

An adoptive cell therapy uses tumor-infiltrating lymphocytes (TILs), a type of lymphocyte found in tumors that are often related to good clinical outcomes. For example, TILs numbers were significantly associated with the prognosis of HCC patients [18]. TIL immunotherapeutic agents can be generated by *ex vivo* expansion of TILs obtained from tumor fragments or digests with IL-2 containing medium for 14 days following activation with anti-CD3 antibody and irradiated allogenic PBMCs [19]. A prior clinical trial demonstrated a better clinical outcome was achieved by TIL compared to lymphokine-activated killer (LAK) cells in advanced melanoma patients. Unfortunately, TILs in HCC were only partially activated, proliferated only at a very low level, acted in an MHC-restricted manner, and consequently failed to effectively kill tumor cells [20].

5.3.2 *Dendritic Cells*

Studies into adoptive immunotherapy involving dendritic cells (DCs) pulsed by tumor lysate or antigens were also undertaken. In the cell-mediated immune response, DCs stimulate the proliferation and activation of antigen-specific cytotoxic T cells and, as such, demonstrating the potency of these professional antigen-presenting cells. To increase the body's immunity against antigens, DCs display large amounts of MHC I and II molecules, costimulatory molecules and stimulatory cytokines (interferon-γ, IL-12) that contribute to an optimal costimulatory environment [21]. This clearly points to the use of autologous DCs as a tumor vaccine, which has been attempted in several cancers including melanoma, prostate cancer, and renal cell carcinoma. In patients with advanced HCC, DCs pulsed *ex vivo* with a HCC cell line lysate were used intravenously in a phase II trial and showed evidence of antitumor efficacy [22]. In HCC patients immunized with DCs pulsed with four alpha-fetoprotein (AFP) peptides as the immunogenic tumor-associated antigen (TAA) instead of tumor cell lysates in phase I/II trials, strong T-cell responses against AFP were noted. Despite this, treated patients did not show clinical responses [23]. Recently, we used an adjuvant autologous DC vaccine pulsed with cytoplasmic transduction peptide (CTP)-attached to three representative TAAs (i.e., alpha-fetoprotein [AFP], glypican-3 [GPC-3] and melanoma-associated antigen 1

[MAGE-1]) in a phase I/IIa study [24]. In that study, patients who did not experience tumor recurrence showed a higher lymphocyte proliferation rate and function than those who experienced recurrence. The patients treated with a DC vaccine showed significantly prolonged median time-to-progression compared to the historical control (36.6 vs 11.8 months). This has led to an ensuing completed phase IIb trial. In phase IIB trial, TAA-pulsed DC vaccine failed to prolong recurrence-free survival in overall patients, although DC vaccine marginally reduced the tumor recurrence in patients who underwent surgical resection [25]. Currently in progress is a multicenter phase III trial in HCC patients who previously underwent surgical resection.

5.3.3 Natural Killer Cells

NK cells kill cells that are dangerous to the host, such as cancer cells or virus-infected cells, and are regarded as key effector cells in cancer immune-surveillance and early viral immunity. Inhibitory receptors for MHC class I molecules (i.e., killer immunoglobulin-like receptors [KIR] and CD94-NKG2A heterodimers) are found on NK cells. The body's immune tolerance for its own tissues occurs when NK cells interact with self MHC class I molecules [26]. In spite of this, the expression of MHC class I molecules on the surface of transformed malignant cells is often reduced resulting the disappearance of inhibitory signaling in NK cells. However, the surface of tumor cells can harbor stress-induced ligands that can be recognized by the activating receptors of NK cells, CD226, NKp44, NKp46, NKp30 and NKG2D. NK cells kill tumor cells mainly via granzyme/perforin activity and sometimes by death-receptor pathways. Additionally, the low-affinity activating receptor, CD16, binds the Fc portion of immunoglobulin G1 and mediates antibody-dependent cellular cytotoxicity.

As an adoptive immunotherapy, both autologous (from the patient) and allogeneic (from a healthy donor) NK cells obtained from peripheral blood have been utilized. Interestingly, allogeneic NK cell therapy led to a higher graft-versus-leukemia effect compared to autologous NK cell therapy for patients with acute myeloid leukemia. Since interaction between self-MHC class I molecules (especially HLA-C) with the KIRs of autologous NK cells can mediate inhibitory signals to NK cells, autologous NK cells may be a more potent source for NK cell immunotherapy. Obtaining sufficient numbers of NK cells to transfer, and maintaining their concentration after transfer have been major hurdles preventing significant clinical effects. Our group is now participating in trials to establish an *ex vivo* expanded and highly activated allogeneic NK cell immunotherapeutic agent from a universal healthy donor. In a phase I trial, allogeneic NK cells derived from unrelated random healthy donors were safely transferred to patients with malignant lymphoma or recurrent solid tumors [27]. A multicenter phase IIa clinical trial to evaluate the efficacy and safety of allogeneic NK cells in patients with intermediate-stage HCC after transarterial chemoembolization (TACE) has recently been launched in Korea (ClinicalTrial.gov ID: NCT02854839).

5.3.4 Lymphokine-Activated Killer Cells

LAK cells were initially described in the early 1980s. Five days of the culture of peripheral blood mononuclear cells (PBMCs) or splenocytes in the presence of IL-2 resulted in the generation of LAK cells, and the killing of tumor cells by effector cells was confirmed *in vitro*.[21] In tumor-bearing mice and patients, LAK cells infused in conjunction with *in vivo* IL-2 co-administration showed anti-tumor activity. However, the induction of severe, IL-2–related toxicities including pulmonary capillary leak syndrome that were dependent on the IL-2 dose, limited the clinical use of LAK cells. When LAK cells were infused without IL-2 treatment, there was minimal toxicity to the recipient but no significant anti-tumor effect. In a murine immunotherapy protocol using LAK cells, splenocytes were used as the source of these cells. In a human clinical trial protocol, repeated leukapheresis was utilized to obtain LAK cells, but it was difficult to generate sufficient cells to transfer. That low proliferation rate of LAK cells was also another hurdle for the clinical use of LAK cells. An adequate anti-tumor response may be achieved from 2×10^{11} human LAK cells as calculated from a murine immunotherapy model, but is difficult to achieve. Other limitations include the ability of exogenous IL-2 to increase cell numbers and the cytolytic activity of LAK cells grown *in vitro* being quite low [28].

5.3.5 Cytokine-Induced Killer Cells

In the late 1980s, anti-CD3 stimulating antibodies was shown to be mitogenic for T lymphocytes. In addition, prolonged culturing also contributed to improving the properties of LAK cells. The cell numbers of human PBMCs increased 300- to 1000-fold when cultured for 2 weeks with both IL-2 and anti-CD3 antibody (OKT3). Under both *in vitro* and *in vivo* conditions, such anti-CD3/IL-2-stimulated human PBMCs were cytolytic for several types of tumor cells in an MHC-unrestricted manner. On closer examination, heterogeneous cells made up the cell population: $CD3^+CD56^+$ NK-like T cells, $CD3^-CD56^+$ NK cells, and $CD3^+CD56^-$ T cells [29]. And because they were stimulated by anti-CD3 and IL-2, such cells were labeled cytokine-induced killer (CIK) cells. In a severe combined immunodeficiency (SCID) mouse model, strong anti-tumor activity was shown by CIK cells against various solid and hematopoietic tumors [30]. In clinical trials, CIK cells exhibited modest tumor killing efficacy against metastatic renal cell carcinoma and melanoma. CIK cells had a higher proliferation ability similar to $CD3^+$ T cells and superior cytolytic activity over LAK cells. Moreover, CIK cells demonstrated potent *in vivo* cytotoxic activity without the need for IL-2 co-administration, which was the major problem in the clinical application of LAK immunotherapy. Considering the lack of a sufficient number of effector cells is one of the substantial hurdles preventing the clinical application of adoptive immunotherapies, a high proliferation rate without toxic IL-2 administration may be a clinically relevant property of CIK cells.

Among the heterogeneous CIK cell population, less than 2% are $CD3^-CD56^+$ NK cells and more than 90% are $CD3^+$ cells, of which up to 35% are $CD56^+$ cells. Similar to NK cells, the anti-tumor activity shown by $CD3^-CD56^+$ cells increases when HLA class I molecules on their target cells are blocked. Tumor cells are more susceptible to being killed by $CD3^+CD56^+$ NK-like T cells than $CD3^+CD56^-$ cells for the following reasons: (i) the presence of a high proportion of $CD8^+$ cells, and (ii) having a more terminally differentiated T cell nature, as well as (iii) a higher granzyme content. More importantly, while $CD3^+CD56^-$ cells are MHC-restricted, the identification and killing of tumor cells by $CD3^+CD56^+$ cells is MHC unrestricted, making the latter pivotal effector CIK cells in tumor killing. Similar to NK cells, which do not require prior sensitization, tumor cells are detected by $CD3^+CD56^+$ cells by the recognition of the cognate ligands, MHC class I polypeptide-related sequences (MIC)-A and -B in an NKG2D-mediated manner (Fig. 5.2). MHC-T-cell receptor (TCR) interaction is not required for the activation of CIK cells by tumor cells. Instead, CIK cells express leukocyte function-associated antigen-1 (LFA-1) that is involved in the identification of tumor cells by these cells and which leads to their stable conjugation. This means that CIK cell immunotherapy is highly relevant for tumor cells expressing LFA-1 ligands including intracellular adhesion molecules (ICAM)-1, -2, and -3. Unsurprisingly, cytolytic activity induced by CIK cells was inhibited by anti-LFA-1 inhibitors.

For normal bone marrow cells *in vitro*, CIK cells show little or no cytotoxicity and thus are markedly tumor specific.

5.4 Adjuvant Cytokine-Induced Killer Cell Immunotherapy for HCC

Studies using *in vitro* and *in vivo* models showed that CIK cells decreased tumor growth [31]. PBMCs expanded *ex vivo* in medium lacking interferon-γ, but when containing anti-CD3 antibody and IL-2 for 14 days developed into CIK cells. In an *in vitro* study of CIK cells, using an effector-target ratio of 30:1 caused 33% of SNU-354 (HCC) cells to die. CIK cells also decreased tumor growth by 60% in a murine HCC model derived from the injection of SNU-354 cells in irradiated nude mice. Mice treated with 1×10^6 or 1×10^7 cells did not show a difference in growth inhibition, which was comparable to treatment with 2 mg/kg of adriamycin. The tumor mass showed a localization of CIK cells *in vivo* and were repeatedly administered without any apparent major adverse events.

In HCC patients who underwent surgical resection in a controlled randomized trial in Japan, the time to disease recurrence was significantly increased after

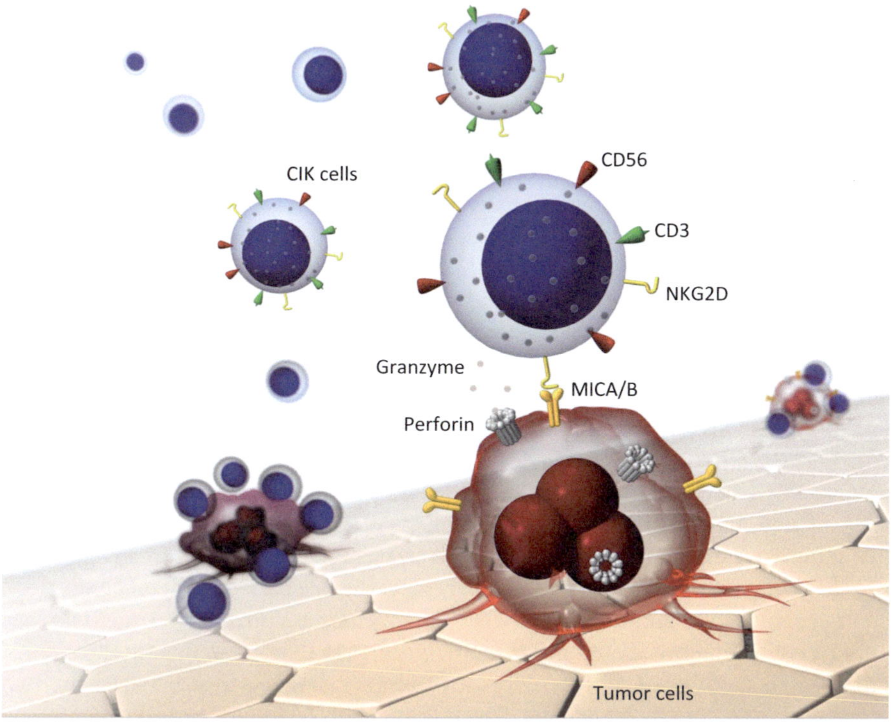

Fig. 5.2 Mechanisms of CD3⁺CD56⁺ cell–induced tumor cell apoptosis. Tumor cells express the cognate ligands, MIC-A and MIC-B, which are recognized by $CD3^+CD56^+$ cells in an NKG2D-dependent manner. After recognition, $CD3^+CD56^+$ cells induce apoptosis of tumor cells using perforin and granzyme

adoptive immunotherapy, with the risk of tumor recurrence decreased by 40% and no difference in overall survival [32]. However, there was no significant difference in overall survival between 74 control patients and 76 treated with CIK cells.

In a Chinese study of HCC, 85 patients were randomized to an immunotherapy or control group after TACE or radiofrequency ablation (RFA) [33]. After CIK cells were injected via the hepatic artery, the peripheral blood showed significant increases in the proportions of $CD3^+$, $CD4^+$, and $CD3^+CD56^+$ cells. The CIK cell treated group showed a significantly lower HCC recurrence compared to the control group (8.9% vs. 30.0%) after 12 months. Only grade 1/2 adverse events were noted for CIK cell therapy.

In another Chinese randomized controlled trial, 127 HCC patients after radical resection were randomized to a CIK cell immunotherapy (three or six cycles) or control group [34]. Undergoing either three or six cycles of CIK cells showed significantly longer disease-free survival than the control group. However, disease-free survival was not different between the three- and six-cycle groups. Multivariate analysis was performed and revealed that treatment with CIK cells was an independent negative predictor of tumor recurrence after adjusting for variables such as vascular invasion, liver cirrhosis and tumor differentiation and size. No survival gain was achieved by CIK cell adjuvant therapy.

Encouraged by these preceding preclinical and clinical studies, the manufacturing process was refined and standardized, and individualized autologous CIK cell-based immunotherapeutic agents were developed. We then sought to examine whether treatment with such adjuvant CIK cells could prolong recurrence-free survival in stage I or II HCC patients after potentially curative treatment (i.e. percutaneous ethanol injection [PEI], RFA, or surgical resection) in a multicenter randomized controlled phase III trial [35]. Two hundred and thirty patients were randomized in equal numbers to immunotherapy or control groups. Patients in the immunotherapy group had 120 mL of blood collected before treatment. The CIK cell agent was manufactured at a central facility. Mononuclear cells were separated and cultured for 2–3 weeks with IL-2 and stimulating monoclonal antibody to CD3 at 37 °C. The CIK cell agent contained a total of 6.4 (±2.1) × 10^9 cells, including 1.8 (±1.0) × 10^9 CIK cells, in 200 mL of fluid. Patients in the immunotherapy group received CIK cell agent intravenously over 60 min and were then observed for at least 30 min. Patients received four treatments of CIK cell agent once a week, and thereafter four treatments every 2, 4 and 8 weeks for a total of 16 treatments. The primary endpoint was recurrence-free survival, with secondary endpoints of safety, and cancer-specific and overall survival. The median recurrence-free survival was 14.0 months longer in the immunotherapy group (44.0 months) than in the control group (30.0 months). The difference in recurrence-free survival between the two groups was statistically significant. The risk of death from tumors or its recurrence decreased by 37% with CIK immunotherapy (Fig. 5.3a). Interestingly, immunotherapy consistently decreased the risk of all types of tumor recurrence: intrahepatic local recurrence (within 2 cm from resection or ablation margin), intrahepatic distant recurrence (beyond 2 cm from margin), and extrahepatic recurrence. In multivariate analysis, CIK cell immunotherapy was a significant prognostic factor after adjustment for age, serum level of serum alpha-fetoprotein, and curative treatment modality. Subgroup analyses showed a beneficial effect on recurrence-free survival for adjuvant therapy compared with no adjuvant treatment, regardless of sex, age, the modality of prior curative treatment, stage of HCC, HCC size, underlying etiology of liver disease, the presence of cirrhosis, and antiviral treatment for HBV (Fig. 5.4). CIK cell immunotherapy also prolonged overall survival: immunotherapy reduced the risk of overall death by 79% (Fig. 5.3b). The immunotherapy group showed significantly longer cancer-specific survival and decreased the risk of HCC-related death by 81%. The immunotherapy group experienced more frequent adverse events but treatment groups did not show a difference in the frequency of grade 3 or 4 adverse events. Common adverse events such as headache (1%), fatigue (3%), chills (8%) and pyrexia (9%) did not contribute to delayed or discontinued CIK cell therapy.

The use of a CIK cell agent in this study was convincingly shown to improve cancer-specific, overall and recurrence-free survival. Although the magnitude of

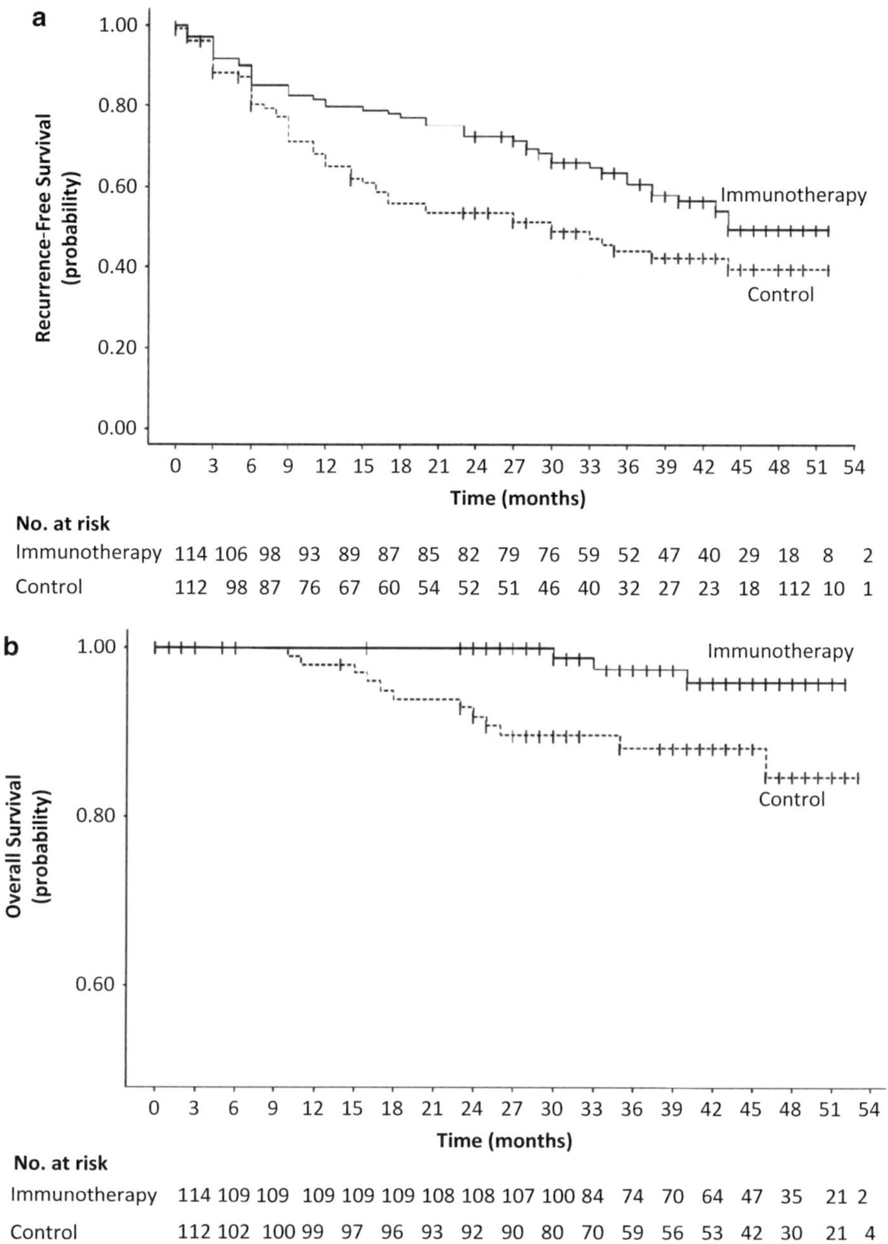

Fig. 5.3 Kaplan-Meier estimates of (**a**) recurrence-free survival and (**b**) overall survival (Reprinted by permission from Elsevier: (GASTROENTEROLOGY) [35], copyright (2015))

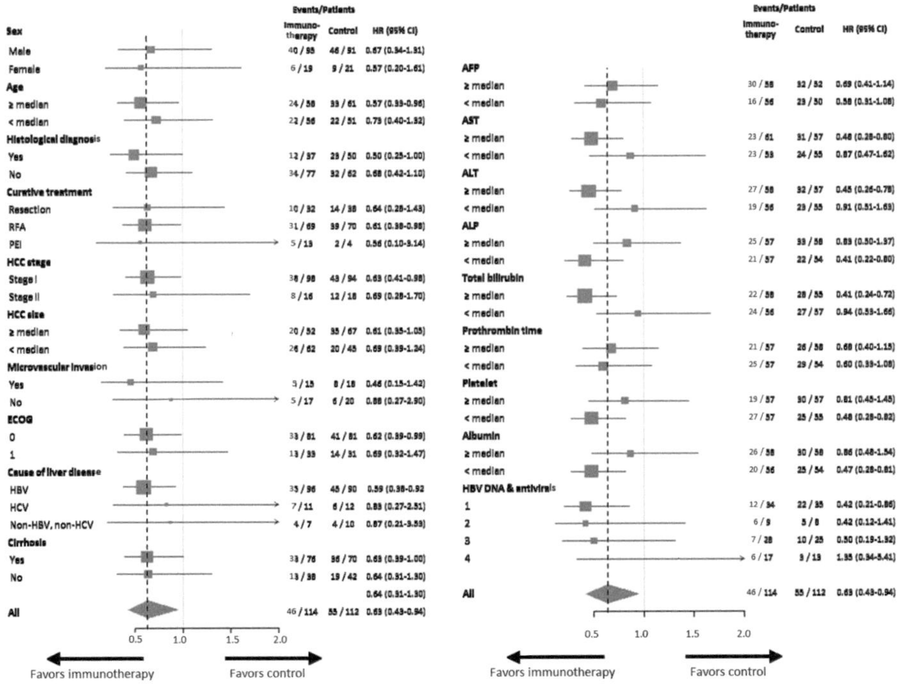

Fig. 5.4 Recurrence-free survival in selected subsets. *Squares* (size proportional to the information quantity) indicate hazard ratio (HR) estimates for each subgroup. *Horizontal lines* represent 95% CIs determined using a Cox proportional hazards model. The line of no effect is represented by a solid *vertical line* at the HR of unity. *Diamonds* represent HRs with 95% CIs for all patients. A *decrease* in the risk of recurrence or death after immunotherapy are represented by HR values less than unity. The HCV subset includes patients co-infected with HBV and HCV. Patients whose serum HBV-DNA levels were ≥2000 IU/mL and who did or did not undergo antiviral treatment are represented by HBV DNA and antiviral agent groups 1 and 2, respectively. Patients whose serum HBV-DNA levels were <2000 IU/mL and who did or did not undergo antiviral treatment are represented by HBV DNA and antiviral agent groups 3 and 4, respectively
AFP α-fetoprotein, *ALP* alkaline phosphatase, *ALT* alanine aminotransferase, *AST* aspartate aminotransferase, *ECOG* Eastern Cooperative Oncology Group, *HCV* hepatitis C virus (Reprinted by permission from Elsevier: (GASTROENTEROLOGY) [35], copyright (2015))

absolute gain was modest, the reduction in relative risk was significant: an approximately 30% reduction in tumor recurrence or death and 80% in both overall and cancer-related mortalities. In particular, CIK cell therapy showed a significant gain in overall survival as well as recurrence-free survival. The intensified schedule of CIK cell agent administration and favorable tumor characteristics in our study may account for the prolonged overall survival observed as compared to prior studies. CIK cells were infused more times (16 times) in our study than in preceding studies (3–10 times). Our study also included only patients with American Joint Committee on Cancer (AJCC) stage I or II hepatocellular carcinoma, whereas preceding studies included patients with a more advanced tumor stage (i.e. stage III or IV tumor, tumor with vascular invasion, or large HCC). Patients with a greater tumor burden in preceding studies may have had increased numbers of immune suppressor cells (e.g. MDSC, T_{reg}s) that attenuated the effect of adjuvant immunotherapy [36, 37], and thus may have impeded any survival benefit.

5.5 Current Limitations of CIK Cell Immunotherapy

CIK cell immunotherapy has several limitations. The expansion rate of CIK cells varies among patients according to the degree of immune suppression. MDSCs and defective APCs can inhibit CIK cell expansion. The quality and quantity of T cells is poor in cancer patients. A lack of reliable serum or histological biomarkers for predicting outcomes of CIK immunotherapy is also a problem. Potential biomarkers include the CD4/CD8 ratio and the proportion of NK cells increase after infusion of CIK cells. Inhibitory immune checkpoints and immune suppressor cells may also be related to the prognosis of patients treated with CIK cells; all these factors that impact CIK cell therapy need to be studied further. In addition, among heterogeneous cells included in CIK cell preparations, most potent effector cells with a high level of NKG2D expression and interferon-γ production are prone to apoptosis, which could limit the prolonged efficacy of CIK cell treatment.

5.6 Future Perspectives

As previously mentioned, adjuvant immunotherapy with autologous CIK cells has been proven to significantly prolong both recurrence-free and overall survival. Several potential methods should be considered to improve the efficacy of CIK cell therapy. Firstly, a combination with different types of adoptive immunotherapy (e.g., combination with adoptive TAA-pulsed DC vaccine) should be considered. Since CIK cells also include a number of cytotoxic T cells that have MHC-restricted cytotoxicity and DCs can provide high levels of MHC I and tumor antigens, a synergistic effect of combination therapy would be expected. Secondly, combination therapy with immune checkpoint inhibitors, such as anti–PD-1/PD-L1 agents and anti–cytotoxic T-lymphocyte–associated protein 4 (CTLA4) agents, may be used to circumvent immune evasion by cancer cells and to stimulate antitumor activity. A recent *in vitro* study reported that blockade of immune checkpoints (including PD-1, KIR, lymphocyte activation gene-3 [LAG-3], and T cell immunoglobulin and mucin-domain-containing-3 [TIM-3]) enhance cytotoxicity of CIK cells against human myeloid leukemic blasts [38]. Thirdly, CIK cells may be stimulated by an increase in MIC-A and -B levels, which bind to NKG2D. The expression of MIC-A and -B can be increased in an epigenetic manner by histone deacetylase inhibitors such as valproic acid and suberoylanilide hydroxamic acid; therefore, combination therapy with these should be considered. Lastly, the downregulation of immune suppressor cells could be helpful in potentiating CIK cell immunotherapy. Low-dose cyclophosphamide treatment was shown to attenuate T_{reg}s [39] and blockade of the signal transducer and activator of transcription 3 (STAT3) suppressed MDSCs [40].

If the efficacy of CIK cell immunotherapy can be maximally potentiated, an investigation of whether CIK cell immunotherapy with/without loco-regional therapy (e.g., TACE) or systemic therapy (e.g., sorafenib) is effective for intermediate or advanced stage HCC may be required. Because maximal tumor reduction before or during adoptive immunotherapy could reduce immune suppressor cells, combination with loco-regional therapy or systemic therapy may allow CIK cells to fight residual tumor cells. In addition, ablation therapies (e.g., RFA) can induce tumor-specific immune responses, which may suggest these could potential combination partners with adoptive immunotherapy [41]. However, combination therapy with CIK cell immunotherapy and sorafenib remains a debatable issue since sorafenib has been reported to impair the function of DCs, tumor-specific T cells, and NK cells, and to increase MDSCs [42–44].

5.7 Conclusion

As an adjuvant therapy after potentially curative treatment for HCC, adoptive immunotherapy using *ex vivo* expanded autologous CIK cells is the only treatment that has been proven to prolong recurrence-free survival as well as overall survival, except for antiviral treatment of HBV-related HCC. The safety of CIK cell immunotherapy has been well demonstrated. However, the clinical efficacy of CIK cells has been shown to exist only for very early or early HCC after curative treatment. Theoretically, maximal tumor reduction before or during adoptive immunotherapy could enhance the efficacy of CIK cells. Combination treatment with other types of adoptive immunotherapy and/or immune checkpoint inhibitors may also potentiate CIK cell therapy.

References

1. Park JW, Chen M, Colombo M, Roberts LR, Schwartz M, Chen PJ, et al. Global patterns of hepatocellular carcinoma management from diagnosis to death: the BRIDGE Study. Liver Int. 2015;35:2155–66.
2. Llovet JM, Di Bisceglie AM, Bruix J, Kramer BS, Lencioni R, Zhu AX, et al. Design and endpoints of clinical trials in hepatocellular carcinoma. J Natl Cancer Inst. 2008;100:698–711.
3. Cho EJ, Lee JH, Yoo JJ, Choi WM, Lee MJ, Cho Y, et al. Serum insulin-like growth factor-I level is an independent predictor of recurrence and survival in early hepatocellular carcinoma: a prospective cohort study. Clin Cancer Res. 2013;19:4218–27.
4. Youn HG, An JY, Choi MG, Noh JH, Sohn TS, Kim S. Recurrence after curative resection of early gastric cancer. Ann Surg Oncol. 2010;17:448–54.

5. Lai EC, Fan ST, Lo CM, Chu KM, Liu CL, Wong J. Hepatic resection for hepatocellular carcinoma. An audit of 343 patients. Ann Surg. 1995;221:291–8.
6. Bruix J, Sherman M, American Association for the Study of Liver D. Management of hepatocellular carcinoma: an update. Hepatology. 2011;53:1020–2.
7. European Association for The Study of The Liver, European Organisation for Research Treatment of Cancer. EASL-EORTC clinical practice guidelines: management of hepatocellular carcinoma. J Hepatol. 2012;56:908–43.
8. Yee C, Greenberg P. Modulating T-cell immunity to tumours: new strategies for monitoring T-cell responses. Nat Rev Cancer. 2002;2:409–19.
9. Bowen DG, Zen M, Holz L, Davis T, McCaughan GW, Bertolino P. The site of primary T cell activation is a determinant of the balance between intrahepatic tolerance and immunity. J Clin Invest. 2004;114:701–12.
10. Thomson AW, Knolle PA. Antigen-presenting cell function in the tolerogenic liver environment. Nat Rev Immunol. 2010;10:753–66.
11. Kuniyasu Y, Marfani SM, Inayat IB, Sheikh SZ, Mehal WZ. Kupffer cells required for high affinity peptide-induced deletion, not retention, of activated CD8+ T cells by mouse liver. Hepatology. 2004;39:1017–27.
12. Grivennikov SI, Greten FR, Karin M. Immunity, inflammation, and cancer. Cell. 2010;140:883–99.
13. Ungefroren H, Sebens S, Seidl D, Lehnert H, Hass R. Interaction of tumor cells with the microenvironment. Cell Commun Signal. 2011;9:18.
14. Zamarron BF, Chen W. Dual roles of immune cells and their factors in cancer development and progression. Int J Biol Sci. 2011;7:651–8.
15. Korangy F, Hochst B, Manns MP, Greten TF. Immune responses in hepatocellular carcinoma. Dig Dis. 2010;28:150–4.
16. Dunn GP, Old LJ, Schreiber RD. The immunobiology of cancer immunosurveillance and immunoediting. Immunity. 2004;21:137–48.
17. Flecken T, Spangenberg HC, Thimme R. Immunobiology of hepatocellular carcinoma. Langenbeck's Arch Surg. 2012;397:673–80.
18. Chew V, Tow C, Teo M, Wong HL, Chan J, Gehring A, et al. Inflammatory tumour microenvironment is associated with superior survival in hepatocellular carcinoma patients. J Hepatol. 2010;52:370–9.
19. Dudley ME, Wunderlich JR, Shelton TE, Even J, Rosenberg SA. Generation of tumor-infiltrating lymphocyte cultures for use in adoptive transfer therapy for melanoma patients. J Immunother. 2003;26:332–42.
20. Rosenberg SA, Spiess P, Lafreniere R. A new approach to the adoptive immunotherapy of cancer with tumor-infiltrating lymphocytes. Science. 1986;233:1318–21.
21. Steinman DA, Rutt BK. On the nature and reduction of plaque-mimicking flow artifacts in black blood MRI of the carotid bifurcation. Magn Reson Med. 1998;39:635–41.
22. Palmer DH, Midgley RS, Mirza N, Torr EE, Ahmed F, Steele JC, et al. A phase II study of adoptive immunotherapy using dendritic cells pulsed with tumor lysate in patients with hepatocellular carcinoma. Hepatology. 2009;49:124–32.
23. Butterfield LH, Ribas A, Dissette VB, Lee Y, Yang JQ, De la Rocha P, et al. A phase I/II trial testing immunization of hepatocellular carcinoma patients with dendritic cells pulsed with four alpha-fetoprotein peptides. Clin Cancer Res. 2006;12:2817–25.
24. Lee JH, Lee Y, Lee M, Heo MK, Song JS, Kim KH, et al. A phase I/IIa study of adjuvant immunotherapy with tumour antigen-pulsed dendritic cells in patients with hepatocellular carcinoma. Br J Cancer. 2015;113:1666–76.
25. Lee JH, Tak WY, Lee Y, Heo MK, Song JS, Kim HY, et al. Adjuvant immunotherapy with autologous dendritic cells for hepatocellualr carcinoma, randomized phase II study. Oncoimmunology. 2017;
26. Raulet DH, Vance RE. Self-tolerance of natural killer cells. Nat Rev Immunol. 2006;6:520–31.

27. Yang Y, Lim O, Kim TM, Ahn YO, Choi H, Chung H, et al. Phase I study of random healthy donor-derived allogeneic natural killer cell therapy in patients with malignant lymphoma or advanced solid tumors. Cancer Immunol Res. 2016;4:215–24.
28. Ahmadzadeh M, Rosenberg SA. IL-2 administration increases CD4+ CD25(hi) Foxp3+ regulatory T cells in cancer patients. Blood. 2006;107:2409–14.
29. Ochoa AC, Gromo G, Alter BJ, Sondel PM, Bach FH. Long-term growth of lymphokine-activated killer (LAK) cells: role of anti-CD3, beta-IL 1, interferon-gamma and -beta. J Immunol. 1987;138:2728–33.
30. Thanendrarajan S, Nowak M, Abken H, Schmidt-Wolf IG. Combining cytokine-induced killer cells with vaccination in cancer immunotherapy: more than one plus one? Leuk Res. 2011;35:1136–42.
31. Kim HM, Lim J, Yoon YD, Ahn JM, Kang JS, Lee K, et al. Anti-tumor activity of ex vivo expanded cytokine-induced killer cells against human hepatocellular carcinoma. Int Immunopharmacol. 2007;7:1793–801.
32. Takayama T, Sekine T, Makuuchi M, Yamasaki S, Kosuge T, Yamamoto J, et al. Adoptive immunotherapy to lower postsurgical recurrence rates of hepatocellular carcinoma: a randomised trial. Lancet. 2000;356:802–7.
33. Weng DS, Zhou J, Zhou QM, Zhao M, Wang QJ, Huang LX, et al. Minimally invasive treatment combined with cytokine-induced killer cells therapy lower the short-term recurrence rates of hepatocellular carcinomas. J Immunother. 2008;31:63–71.
34. Hui D, Qiang L, Jian W, Ti Z, Da-Lu K. A randomized, controlled trial of postoperative adjuvant cytokine-induced killer cells immunotherapy after radical resection of hepatocellular carcinoma. Dig Liver Dis. 2009;41:36–41.
35. Lee JH, Lee JH, Lim YS, Yeon JE, Song TJ, Yu SJ, et al. Adjuvant immunotherapy with autologous cytokine-induced killer cells for hepatocellular carcinoma. Gastroenterology. 2015;148:1383–91. e6
36. Beyer M, Schultze JL. Regulatory T cells in cancer. Blood. 2006;108:804–11.
37. Diaz-Montero CM, Salem ML, Nishimura MI, Garrett-Mayer E, Cole DJ, Montero AJ. Increased circulating myeloid-derived suppressor cells correlate with clinical cancer stage, metastatic tumor burden, and doxorubicin-cyclophosphamide chemotherapy. Cancer Immunol Immunother. 2009;58:49–59.
38. Poh SL, Linn YC. Immune checkpoint inhibitors enhance cytotoxicity of cytokine-induced killer cells against human myeloid leukaemic blasts. Cancer Immunol Immunother. 2016;65:525–36.
39. Greten TF, Ormandy LA, Fikuart A, Hochst B, Henschen S, Horning M, et al. Low-dose cyclophosphamide treatment impairs regulatory T cells and unmasks AFP-specific CD4+ T-cell responses in patients with advanced HCC. J Immunother. 2010;33:211–8.
40. Vasquez-Dunddel D, Pan F, Zeng Q, Gorbounov M, Albesiano E, Fu J, et al. STAT3 regulates arginase-I in myeloid-derived suppressor cells from cancer patients. J Clin Invest. 2013;123:1580–9.
41. Greten TF, Duffy AG, Korangy F. Hepatocellular carcinoma from an immunologic perspective. Clin Cancer Res. 2013;19:6678–85.
42. Hipp MM, Hilf N, Walter S, Werth D, Brauer KM, Radsak MP, et al. Sorafenib, but not sunitinib, affects function of dendritic cells and induction of primary immune responses. Blood. 2008;111:5610–20.
43. Chen Y, Huang Y, Reiberger T, Duyverman AM, Huang P, Samuel R, et al. Differential effects of sorafenib on liver versus tumor fibrosis mediated by stromal-derived factor 1 alpha/C-X-C receptor type 4 axis and myeloid differentiation antigen-positive myeloid cell infiltration in mice. Hepatology. 2014;59:1435–47.
44. Krusch M, Salih J, Schlicke M, Baessler T, Kampa KM, Mayer F, et al. The kinase inhibitors sunitinib and sorafenib differentially affect NK cell antitumor reactivity in vitro. J Immunol. 2009;183:8286–94.

Chapter 6
Anti-VEGFR Therapy as a Partner for Immune-Based Therapy Approaches in HCC

Kohei Shigeta, Tai Hato, Yunching Chen, and Dan G. Duda

6.1 Introduction

Hepatocellular carcinoma (HCC) is the second most common cancer-related cause of death worldwide and a major cause of death in patients with cirrhosis. When curative surgeries (resection or transplant) cannot be performed, therapeutic options are limited. Sorafenib – a multitargeted tyrosine kinase inhibitor (TKI) – was the first drug approved for the systemic therapy of advanced stage HCC. Sorafenib is the worldwide standard of care for advanced HCC patients based on data showing increased overall survival (OS) in phase III trials. However, these studies also showed that HCCs rarely shrink after sorafenib treatment and rapidly become resistant to sorafenib, which limits the OS benefit to less than 3 months. Furthermore, despite aggressive development of other anti-vascular endothelial growth factor receptor (VEGFR) TKIs or antibodies, many of these agents have failed so far to match its efficacy, for reasons that are not clear yet.

More recent developments have brought some promise for the systemic therapy of HCC. A drug related to sorafenib, regorafenib, has shown efficacy in second line setting, in patients with recurrent HCC after sorafenib [1]. Based on this result, regorafenib has recently become the second-line treatment for advanced HCC. In addition, immune checkpoint blockers (ICBs), which have transformed the management of melanoma, and lung and head-and-neck cancers, have also shown promise in the treatment of HCC. Phase III trials of anti-programmed death 1 receptor (PD-1) antibodies are currently ongoing both in first– and second-line setting. Interim results from these trials showed durable responses to IBC therapy in nearly 20% of HCC patients [2].

K. Shigeta • T. Hato • Y. Chen • D.G. Duda (✉)
E.L. Steele Laboratories for Tumor Biology, Department of Radiation Oncology, Massachusetts General Hospital Cancer Center, Harvard Medical School, 100 Blossom St, Cox-734, Boston, MA 02114, USA
e-mail: gduda@partners.org

T.F. Greten (ed.), *Immunotherapy of Hepatocellular Carcinoma*,
DOI 10.1007/978-3-319-64958-0_6

The majority of HCC patients suffer from underlying viral hepatitis (with virus B or C). In these patients, prolonged mild inflammation promotes an immunosuppressive environment in the liver. The failure of the immune system to prevent HCC and to halt its progression is closely linked with the pathogenesis and survival of these cancer patients. Thus, given the promise of ICBs, approaches aimed at boosting HCC-specific immune responses are timely and of great interest currently. In this chapter, we will summarize the current knowledge of immune responses in HCC – with the focus on immune checkpoints – and will discuss the rationale of combining standard anti-VEGFR strategies with emerging ICBs.

6.2 Anti-VEGFR Therapy with Sorafenib for HCC

Sorafenib is a multitargeted drug that inhibits VEGFR1, −2, and −3, as well as platelet-derived growth factor receptor beta (PDGFR-β). Sorafenib was initially developed as an inhibitor of the serine-threonine kinases RAF-1 and B-RAF. The mechanisms of action of this drug are complex and incompletely understood, and may include both inhibition of HCC cell viability, tumor angiogenesis and liver fibrosis [3–5]. The effect of sorafenib on the immune environment of HCC and on the systemic anti-tumor immune responses is incompletely characterized.

Sorafenib became standard treatment for HCC based on data from two global phase III clinical trials: the SHARP trial and the Asia-Pacific study for Child–Pugh A advanced HCC [6, 7]. The SHARP trial was a phase III, double blind, placebo-controlled trial, and 602 patients with advanced HCC who had not received previous systemic treatment were randomly assigned to receive either sorafenib or placebo. Median OS was nearly 3 months longer in sorafenib group comparing to placebo group (10.7 months in the sorafenib and 7.9 months in the placebo group; hazard ratio 0.69; $p < 0.001$). There was no significant difference between the two groups in the median time to symptomatic progression, however the median time to radiologic progression was 5.5 months in the sorafenib group and 2.8 months in the placebo group ($p < 0.001$). Another phase III trial, the Asia-Pacific study, enrolled Asian patients with HCC who had not received previous systemic therapy and had good liver function (Child-Pugh class A). Two hundred and seventy-one patients were randomly assigned to receive either oral sorafenib or placebo. Median OS was 6.5 months in patients treated with sorafenib, compared with 4.2 months in those who received placebo [hazard ratio (HR) = 0.68; p = 0.014]. Median time-to-progression (TTP) was also prolonged in the sorafenib group compared to the placebo group.

Unfortunately, subsequent phase III trials combining sorafenib with other agents have been unsuccessful so far to further prolong OS. For example, combination of sorafenib with the anti-epidermal growth factor receptor (EGFR) TKI erlotinib [8] or with local trans-arterial chemo-embolization (TACE) [9] failed to show increased OS in advanced HCC. Several ongoing clinical trials are evaluating the efficacy of sorafenib combined with other local ablative therapies such as radiofrequency ablation (RFA) or cryoablation.

6.3 Development of Other Targeted Therapies in Advanced HCC

The successful development of sorafenib in HCC prompted a large clinical effort of developing other targeted therapies in this disease, which included randomized phase III trials in first-line and second-line of approved anti-VEGFR drugs or experimental agents. Unfortunately, the therapeutic efficacy of most agents was largely disappointing [10].

Sunitinib, a multikinase inhibitor with broad spectrum of activity blocking VEGFR, PDGFR, and KIT, among other kinases, is a standard of care in several cancers. A randomized phase III trial of sunitinib first-line for advanced HCC (SUN1170 trial) had to be discontinued early owing to the toxicity of sunitinib in this population [11]. The median OS with sunitinib was 7.9 months, which was significantly shorter than in the sorafenib arm (10.2 months).

Everolimus is a mammalian target of rapamycin (mTOR) inhibitor approved for renal cancer. A phase III trial (EVOLVE-1) of everolimus as second-line treatment in advanced HCC failed to show superiority in OS for this drug compared to placebo [12].

Ramucirumab is a recombinant IgG1 monoclonal antibody that has a high affinity for the extracellular domain of VEGFR-2, currently approved for advanced gastric and lung cancer. In a phase III trial (REACH study) of ramucirumab as a second-line treatment for advanced HCC, there was no significant difference in OS between the ramucirumab and placebo group. However, a sub-group analysis showed a significant improvement in OS after ramucirumab in patients with high baseline alpha-fetoprotein (AFP) levels (400 ng/mL or greater) [13]. As a result, a phase III trial (REACH-2) is underway for advanced HCC patients with AFP levels.

Cabozantinib is a multi-kinase inhibitor that inhibits MET, VEGFR-2, and RET, approved for several indications. A phase II trial of cabozantinib in patients with advanced HCC with a history of systemic chemotherapy showed a median PFS was 4.2 months. A phase III trial (CELESTIAL) of cabozantinib as a second-line treatment is currently underway. Recently, after the first planned interim analysis of CELESTIAL data, the trial's Independent Data Monitoring Committee (IDMC) determined that the study should continue without modifications per the study protocol [14].

Brivanib is a dual tyrosine kinase inhibitor of VEGFR and fibroblast growth factor receptors (FGFRs). In a phase II trial of brivanib in HCC, median progression-free survival (PFS) was 2.7 months and median OS was 10 months [15]. A randomized phase III trial of brivanib (BRISK-FL) compared this agent with sorafenib in first-line setting, but the study did not demonstrate the superiority or non-inferiority of brivanib [16]. A second randomized phase III trial of brivanib (BRISK-PS) in second-line setting also failed to show increased OS in sorafenib intolerant or resistant HCC [17].

Linifanib is a TKI against VEGFR and PDGFR. In the randomized phase III trial of linifanib (LIGHT) as a first-line treatment, this drug was neither superior nor non-inferior to sorafenib [18].

Tivantinib is an agent developed as a selective MET inhibitor. In a phase II trial of tivantinib as a second line treatment, time-to-tumor-progression was longer in the tivantinib group than in the placebo group (HR = 0.64; p = 0.04) [19]. However, the sponsor recently announced that the phase III trial (METIV-HCC [20]) of tivantinib as a second line treatment only for patients with high intratumoral c-MET expression did not reach its primary endpoint of improving OS.

The only suuccessful studies in the "post-sorafenib era" were those of a related compound (regorafenib) used in second line setting and of another multikinase inhibitor (lenvatinib) in first line setting. Regorafenib is a multikinase inhibitor that targets VEGFR1–3, KIT, RET, BRAF, PDGFR, and FGFR and is approved for metastatic colorectal cancer and gastrointestinal stromal tumors (GIST). In a phase II trial of regorafenib in patients previously treated with sorafenib, the median OS was 13.8 months (95% CI: 9.3, 18.3), which suggested a good activity [1]. Based on these results, a phase III trial (RESORCE) was initiated to test regorafenib as a second-line treatment. The trial showed that regorafenib significantly increased median OS to 10.6 months compared to 7.8 months for best supportive care (HR = 0.62; $p < 0.001$).

Lenvatinib is a multi-TKI for VEGFR1–3, FGFR1–4, PDGFR, and is rearranged during transfection (RET). Phase I and II trials were conducted for Child–Pugh A advanced HCC resistant to standard treatment [21, 22]. The response rate was 34.8% and the median OS was 18.3 months (95% CI: 12.8, N/A), which was a promising result. Initial results of a phase III trial in first-line treatment in HCC patients (E7080) were recently released. This was a multicenter, randomized, global phase III study comparing the efficacy and safety of lenvatinib versus sorafenib, as a first-line treatment for patients with unresectable HCC. Lenvatinib met the statistical criteria for non-inferiority of OS (13.6 months) compared to sorafenib (12.3 months), and showed statistically significant and clinically meaningful improvement for PFS, TTP and ORR (7.4 months, 8.9 months and 24%). Analyses of the remaining secondary endpoints of quality of life and safety are ongoing [23].

In addition, other studies pursued sorafenib-based combination approaches, such as for example the EGFR TKI erlotinib. A randomized phase III trial with sorafenib + erlotinib versus sorafenib was conducted as a first-line phase III trial (SEARCH trial) for advanced HCC [8]. However, the combination therapy did not show an increase in OS over sorafenib alone.

As a result of this clinical experience, sorafenib remains the only first-line drug for advanced HCC, with the potential implementation of lenvatinib in this setting. Regorafenib is expected to become the second-line of therapy for advanced HCC patients with recurrence after sorafenib.

The advent of ICBs has brought new hope for advanced HCC, but their optimal implementation will require a better understanding of how these drugs affect the tumor microenvironment and systemic immune responses in this disease.

6.4 Mechanisms of Resistance to Sorafenib in HCC and Their Relevance to Immunotherapy

Sorafenib is widely considered as an antiangiogenic/antivascular drug through inhibition of VEGFRs and PDGFRs. However, as discussed above, many potent and/or more selective anti-VEGFR agents or more broad antiangiogenic agents (e.g., VEGFR/FGFR and anti-VEGFR/PDGFR inhibitors) have thus far failed to match the efficacy of sorafenib in phase III trials in HCC. Moreover, antiangiogenic therapy has not led to tumor regression in patients or in experimental models in mice. The benefit noted with sorafenib in HCC patients is likely the result of a transient delay in HCC growth, after which most tumors resume their growth.

Whereas the mechanisms of acquired resistance to sorafenib and other anti-VEGFR inhibitors in HCC remain to be fully characterized, it is likely that tumor stroma-mediated survival pathways and immunosuppression might play key roles. Of these, increased hypoxia has been proposed as a mechanism of resistance to multitargeted TKI therapy. The key is to identify the critical molecular pathways regulating stroma-mediated resistance to sorafenib treatment in HCC.

Hypoxia and other cellular stresses can promote the expression of the chemokine stromal-derived factor 1 alpha (SDF1α) or C-X-C ligand 12 (CXCL12), and of its receptor, C-X-C receptor type 4 (CXCR4). We have previously shown that SDF1α levels increase in plasma circulation in HCC patients after treatment with sunitinib or cediranib (both anti-VEGFR/PDGFR TKIs) in clinical studies. Moreover, elevated circulating levels of SDF1α correlated with poor treatment outcome after sunitinib treatment in HCC patients. Systemic activation of the SDF1α/CXCR4 axis is known to mediate intratumoral infiltration of inflammatory cells, including myeloid differentiation antigen–positive (Gr-1$^+$) myeloid (CD11b$^+$) cells. Gr-1$^+$ myeloid cells can drive tumor recurrence after anti-VEGF therapy in various tumor models. Finally, clinical correlative data also strongly suggested that the effects on multitargeted TKI treatment on tumor vasculature and myeloid cells might mediate response and resistance therapy in HCC patients.

In a recent report, we demonstrated the causal role of Gr-1$^+$ myeloid cells in HCC resistance to antiangiogenic treatment [3]. Furthermore, our preclinical studies provided a mechanistic understanding of the interplay between treatment-induced hypoxia, SDF1α/CXCR4 pathway activation, and Gr-1$^+$ myeloid cell infiltration and tumor fibrosis in HCC. Using an orthotopic model of HCC and liver damage in mice, we evaluated the effect of sorafenib on tumor fibrosis and liver fibrosis. Whereas sorafenib reduced liver fibrosis, its antivascular effects led to increased hypoxia, inflammation, and fibrosis in the tumor tissues, which associated

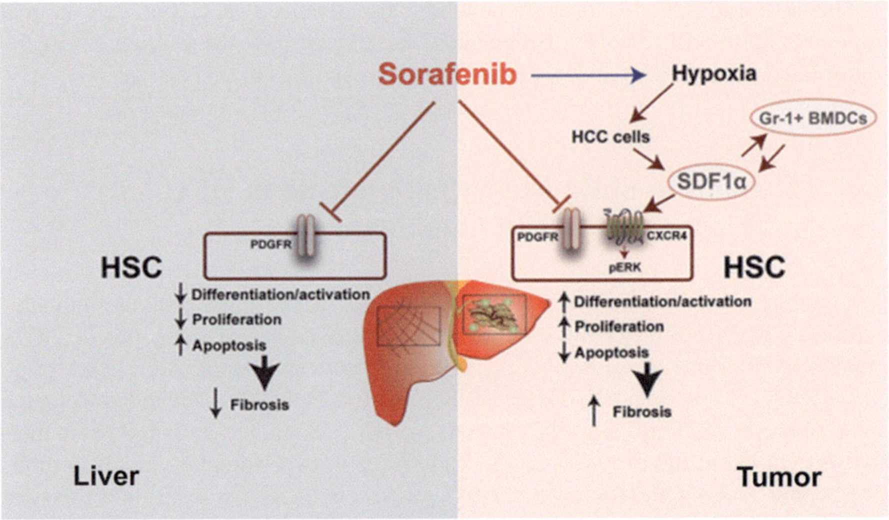

Fig. 6.1 Differential effect of sorafenib on liver versus tumor-associated fibrosis mediated by the SDF-1α/CXCR4 axis and Gr-1⁺ cells in HCC. Differential effects of sorafenib are the result of increased intratumoral hypoxia, leading to elevated SDF-1α expression and Gr-1⁺ myeloid cell infiltration. Blocking CXCR4 prevents Gr-1⁺ myeloid cell infiltration and HSC differentiation and activation, and synergizes with the antitumor effects of sorafenib

with resistance to sorafenib treatment. We also showed that in this context, the pro-fibrotic effects of SDF1α were sufficient to overcome PDGFR inhibition by sorafenib and increased intratumoral fibrosis (Fig. 6.1). SDF1α induced differentiation and proliferation of hepatic stellate cells (HSCs) directly through MAPK activation after sorafenib treatment. More importantly, addition of CXCR4 inhibition to sorafenib treatment prevented the increase in desmoplasia in the face of persistent hypoxia. Moreover, this combination therapy significantly inhibited HCC growth, compared to sorafenib alone.

Increased SDF1α expression can also lead to accumulation of tumor-promoting (proangiogenic and immune-suppressive) inflammatory cells. CXCR4 is known to be critical for myeloid cell infiltration in tumors and can compensate for VEGFR1 inhibition in bone marrow–derived cells, as demonstrated by our group using pharmacologic and genetic models of CXCR4 inhibition [24]. Indeed, we found increased intratumoral infiltration by Gr-1⁺ myeloid cells in HCC after sorafenib treatment. Paracrine interactions between HSCs and inflammatory cells leading to liver fibrosis are also critical in viral hepatitis and pancreatic malignancies. Our studies indicated that the SDF1α/CXCR4 axis plays an important role mediating not only Gr-1⁺ myeloid cell infiltration in HCC, but also their paracrine interaction with HSCs leading to fibrosis. SDF1α expression promoted tumor vascularization, likely by recruitment of proangiogenic Gr-1⁺ myeloid cells. Finally, antibody blockade of Gr-1 reduced Gr-1⁺ myeloid cell infiltration, tumor desmoplasia, and HCC growth.

In addition to proangiogenic and proinflammatory effects, hypoxia can trigger EMT in cancer cells, which may also play an important role in tumor progression and particularly in metastasis. Indeed, CXCR4 blockade prevented EMT despite persistent hypoxia, reduced metastatic burden, and increased survival in mice with HCC. These findings may be relevant not only for sorafenib but also for any other hypoxia-inducing anti-angiogenic therapy in HCC.

6.5 Immune Checkpoint Therapy for HCC

As a typical "inflammation-induced cancer", HCC most frequently develops in a diseased liver. Prolonged inflammation from viral hepatitis induces an immunosuppressive environment in the liver [25, 26]. Based on research with patients with viral hepatitis and mouse models of hepatitis, it is known that cytotoxic T lymphocyte associated antigen 4 (CTLA-4), programmed death 1 (PD-1), mucin domain–containing molecule 3, and 2B4 (CD244) are upregulated and, as a result, $CD8^+$ T cell functioning becomes severely impaired (leading to T cell exhaustion) [27–29]. In addition, dendritic cell (DC) function is also impaired in HCC patients. DC in HCC patients showed a reduced expression of pro-inflammatory cytokines, such as IL-12, which results in defective activation in $CD8^+$ T cells [30]. To make matters worse, increased infiltration by regulatory T cells (Tregs) is frequently seen in HCC [31]. Finally, it has been recently found that myeloid-derived suppressor cells (MDSCs), which are immature cell types of myeloid origin, infiltrate into the tumor and induce increased Treg recruitment in HCC in patients [32].

The success of ICB with anti-CTLA-4 antibodies in advanced melanoma patients has brought renewed hope for immunotherapy in cancer [33]. HCC is typically an inflammation-associated cancer and can be immunogenic. Furthermore, the majority of HCC patients suffer from cirrhosis of viral etiology or nonalcoholic steatohepatitis. Since immunotherapeutic drugs are not metabolized in the liver, they may have predictable pharmacokinetic profiles in cirrhotic patients. Indeed, preliminary clinical data with antibody-based therapy did not show any severe hepatoxicity. Nevertheless, the successful application of immunotherapy in HCC will have to take into account the liver cancer-specific immune microenvironment and responses.

6.6 How Do HCCs Evade Anti-tumor Immunity?

Spontaneous anti-tumor responses have been detected in HCC patients. Activation of immune response and T cell infiltration has been reported after percutaneous ethanol injection or radiofrequency ablation. In addition, tumor-associated antigen (TAA) specific $CD8^+$ T cell immune responses have been described. Among the most studied antigens in HCC are alpha-fetoprotein (AFP), glypican-3 (GPC-3), NY-ESO-1, SSX-2, melanoma antigen gene-A (MAGE-A) and human telomerase-reverse transcriptase (hTERT). One report estimated that more than 50% of HCC patients develop spontaneous cellular or humoral immune response against NY-ESO-1. Another study reported that HCC-infiltrating TAA-specific CD8+ T cells were detectable in more than 50% of patients and their number correlated with progression-free survival.

The immune microenvironment of the liver plays a major role in anti-tumor immunity. Liver is generally "tolerogenic" to prevent undesirable immune response to antigens absorbed from the gut. The tolerability is maintained by direct activation of naïve T cells in liver through antigen presentation by liver sinusoidal endothelial cells, Kuppfer cells, dendritic cells (DCs) and hepatocytes. In addition, intricate immunosuppressive mechanisms become activated in the HCC microenvironment and further interfere with the development of meaningful anti-tumor immune responses. Multiple such mechanisms have been proposed, including defective antigen presentation, recruitment of immunosuppressive myeloid and lymphoid cell populations, suppression of natural killer (NK) cells, impaired $CD4^{+}$ T cell functions, and up-regulation of immune checkpoint pathways.

Among immunosuppressive cell populations, Tregs and MDSCs are thought to play key roles in cancer evasion from immunosurveillance. In HCC, the number of Tregs is increased both in the blood circulation and inside the tumor. Intratumoral Treg accumulation correlates with disease progression and poor prognosis. MDSCs are immature/progenitor myeloid cells with immunosuppressive and pro-angiogenic activity. MDSC accumulation is found not only within the tumors but also in blood circulation, spleen, bone marrow and liver. The MDSCs inhibit the function of effector T cells, decrease NK cell cytotoxicity, and cytokine production. The frequency of MDSCs correlates with recurrence-free survival of HCC patients who underwent RFA. It has also been suggested that MDSCs interact with Kuppfer cells to induce PD-L1 expression, which in turn inhibits antigen presentation. MDSCs may also help expand Treg population. Depletion of Tregs or MDSCs could prompt spontaneous immune responses against AFP, suggesting the potential of immune reactivation. Recently, a new subset of immune suppressive cells called regulatory DCs has been identified in HCC patients. These regulatory DCs can suppress T cell activation through interleukin (IL)-10 and indoleamine 2,3-dioxygenase (IDO) production.

Exhaustion of $CD4^{+}$ T cells has also been reported as a mechanism of immune evasion in HCC. While infrequent AFP-specific CD4+ T cells are detectable in early disease, they became exhausted and fail to execute their immune supportive function once the disease has advanced. Finally, while the immune response to specific antigen is recognized by major histocompatibility receptors, co-stimulatory and co-inhibitory molecules regulate the intensity of response. Immune checkpoints are co-inhibitory molecules that are physiologically expressed for the maintenance of self-tolerance. In the tumor microenvironment, immune checkpoint molecules such as CTLA-4 and PD-L1 are often overexpressed and participate in the evasive mechanism as discussed above.

6.7 Translation of Immune Checkpoint Blockade in HCC

The balance of co-stimulatory signals and immune checkpoints determines the cytotoxic T cell activation and intensity of immune response. The immune checkpoints are often activated in the tumor tissue, which promotes tumor evasion from host immunity. The most studied immune checkpoint receptors are CTLA-4, PD-1, TIM-3, BTLA, VISTA and LAG-3. However, there are still few studies that evaluated the efficacy of combination therapy with sorafenib and ICBs.

6.8 PD-1: Mechanism of Action

PD-1 is CD28 superfamily member that conveys co-inhibitory signals for TCR receptor. PD-1 binds its ligands PD-L1 (CD274) or PD-L2 (CD273). PD-1 is primarily expressed in CD8+ T cells, but can also be detected on Tregs and MDSCs. PD-1 mediates the differentiation and proliferation of Tregs. Interestingly, a recent report by Tian et al. showed that activation of CD4+ T lymphocytes by ICBs (anti-PD-1 and anti-CTLA4) can also promote vascular normalization [34]. PD-1 also regulates peripheral tolerance and autoimmunity. Chronic exposure to antigens leads to the overexpression of PD-1 in T cells, which induces anergy or cell exhaustion. By chronic antigen stimulation, IFN-γ induces IRF9 binding to Pdcd-1 promoter and PD-1 transcription in T cells. When PD-1 binds to PD-L1 or PD-L2, T cell proliferation and cytokine release are inhibited through SHP2, which inactivates ZAP70, a major TCR signaling integrator. T cell function is differentially affected by the level of PD-1 activity. Cancer cells can highjack PD-L1/PD-1 signaling by expressing PD-L1 or PD-L2 to activate PD-1 in tumor-infiltrating lymphocytes and evade immune surveillance.

While the mechanisms of immune tolerance to viral hepatitis are well described, limited data are available for HCC. Two mouse models showed the potential relevance of PD-1/PD-L1 induced immune tolerance in HCC. In a genetic model of c-Myc-induced HCC and doxycycline-induced expression of IL-12 in hepatocytes, doxycycline treatment induced IFN-γ expression but only a partial regression of the tumors. Treatment resistance was associated with increase in Treg numbers and upregulation of several immune checkpoint molecules (including PD-L1/PD-1). In another mouse model of HCC induced by adenovirus-mediated inducible SV40 large T antigen expression in hepatocytes, T cell infiltration into the tumor was decreased in the advanced lesions.

6.9 Clinical Studies of PD-1 Blockade

At least 5 anti-PD-1 antibodies and 3 anti-PD-L1 antibodies are currently under development, emphasizing the growing interest in this immune checkpoint pathway as a target for cancer therapy (Table 6.1) [35]. Pembrolizumab induced tumor regression in advanced melanoma patients and showed a favorable safety profile. Interestingly, pembrolizumab was effective even in patients who failed ipilimumab treatment, which suggests a differential mechanism of action for PD-1 inhibition versus CTLA-4 blockade. Indeed, combination of nivolumab with iplimumab achieved objective response in 40% of the patients with less toxicity. CT-011 and MPDL3280A/RG7446 were tested in phase I trials and showed with favorable safety profiles. MEDI4376 targets PD-L1, and phase I trial is ongoing. AMP-224 is a recombinant B7-DC-Fc fusion protein, and a phase I trial of this agent is also underway. In HCC, a phase I/II trial of CT-011 in advanced HCC was initiated but stopped due to slow accrual. A phase I trial of nivolumab for patients with advanced HCC (NCT01658878) resulted that nivolumab has a manageable AE profile and produced durable responses across all dose levels and HCC cohorts, with a favorable 6-month OS rate. Currently, a phase III trial of first-line treatment nivolumab compared to sorafenib (NCT02576509) is ongoing, and a phase III trial of pembrolizumab versus best supportive care (KEYNOTE-240) is ongoing in second-line setting (NCT02702401) in advanced HCC patients.

6.10 Testing Anti-PD-1 Therapy Combined with Sorafenib in the Preclinical Setting

Due to promiscuous target inhibition by sorafenib, the mechanisms of treatment evasion are likely multifactorial as discussed above. One mechanism may be the increase in tissue hypoxia after prolonged anti-angiogenic therapy, which likely promotes tumor recurrence locally and at distant sites. Hypoxia can fuel resistance to treatment not only by promoting genomic instability, angiogenesis, and invasion but also by creating an immunosuppressive microenvironment. Increased hypoxia results in recruitment and activation of multiple myeloid and lymphoid immune suppressor cells such as M2-type tumor-associated macrophages (TAMs), MDSCs, and Tregs. Increased hypoxia after sorafenib treatment induces SDF1α and CXCR4 expression and myeloid differentiation antigen $Gr\text{-}1^+$ myeloid-derived suppressor cell recruitment. As discussed above, inhibition of the SDF1α/CXCR4 axis prevented the increase in tumor desmoplasia and inhibited tumor growth despite persistent hypoxia.

Table 6.1 Immune checkpoint blocking antibodies and status of clinical development for HCC

Target	Antibody	Trial ID	Phase	Treatment	Status	Results
CTLA-4	Tremelimumab (formerly referred to as ticilimumab, CP-675,206, MedImmune, USA & Pfizer, USA)	NCT01008358	I	Monotherapy	Completed	Well tolerated
						Disease control rate of 76.4%
						Median OS 8.2 month [95%CI: 4.64,21.34]
		NCT01853618	I	In combination with RFA or TACE	Ongoing	N/A
	Ipilimumab (MDX-010, Bristol-Myers Squibb, USA)	NCT01658878	I/II	In combination with or without Nivolumab	Ongoing	Well tolerated
						Disease control rate of 64%
						9-month overall survival rate in the expansion phase was 74%
PD-1	Nivolumab (BMS-936558, Bristol-Myers Squibb, USA)	NCT01658878	I/II	Monotherapy	Ongoing	Well tolerated
						Disease control rate of 46.2%
						Overall survival rate at 6 months is 72%
		NCT02576509	III	Monotherapy	Ongoing	N/A
	CT-011 (CureTech, Israel)	NCT00966251	I/II	Monotherapy	Terminated	Stopped due to slow accrual
	Lambrolizumab/ pembrolizumab (MK-3475, Merck, USA)	NCT02658019	II	Monotherapy	Ongoing	N/A
		NCT02702401	III	Monotherapy	Ongoing	N/A
		NCT03006926	I	Combination with Lenvatinib	Ongoing	N/A
	AMP-224 (Amplimmune, USA)	N/A	N/A	N/A	N/A	N/A
PD-L1	MPDL3280A/RG7446 (Genentech, USA &Roche, Switzerland)	N/A	N/A	N/A	N/A	N/A
	MEDI4736 (MedImmune, USA &AstraZeneca, UK)	NCT02519348	II	Combination with or without Tremelimimab	Ongoing	N/A
		NCT02821754	I/II	In combination with Tremelimumab and RFA or TACE	Ongoing	N/A

Clinical data regarding the presence, infiltration, and function of T-infiltrating lymphocytes in HCC are limited. Case reports and a cohort study report the rare presence of T-infiltrating lymphocytes in human HCCs. Moreover, the presence and function of T-infiltrating lymphocytes may be a prognostic marker in HCC patients. Therefore, a combination of depletion of Tregs and concomitant stimulation of effector T cells may represent an effective strategy to reduce HCC metastasis and recurrence. PD-1 blockade has been successfully used for the treatment of late-stage melanoma and in other solid tumors, however achieving similar efficacy with ICBs in HCC will largely depend on how they are integrated with sorafenib. For example, it has also been recently shown that cancer cells, cancer-associated stromal cells, and a hypoxic tumor microenvironment can up-regulate immune regulatory proteins (PD-L1 or its receptor PD-1) that facilitate tumor escape from immune surveillance. Up-regulation of PD-L1/PD-1 inhibits cytotoxic $CD8^+$ T-lymphocyte activation and proliferation and further contributes to resistance and progression of solid tumors.

We used orthotopic (grafted and genetically engineered) murine models of HCC to examine the role of PD-1 blockade on primary tumor growth, lung metastasis, and the immune microenvironment after sorafenib treatment. In addition to $Gr\text{-}1^+$ myeloid cells, there was an increase in M2-type TAMs and Tregs infiltrated in tumors after sorafenib treatment, indicating the induction of an immunosuppressive microenvironment in sorafenib-treated HCCs. CXCR4 blockade reduced the infiltration of these immunosuppressive cells despite persistent hypoxia but failed to promote antitumor cellular immune responses. This preclinical study demonstrated that anti-PD-1 immunotherapy was active against both grafted and spontaneous tumors. However, anti-PD-1 blockade did not significantly delay tumor growth or metastasis when combined with sorafenib, likely owing to the increased immunosuppression after sorafenib treatment. Sorafenib plus anti-PD-1 antibody significantly delayed HCC growth and reduced lung metastasis only when combined with anti-CXCR4 therapy. Triple combination treatment was safe and associated with increased tumor penetration by activated $CD8^+$ T lymphocytes and accompanying increased HCC cell apoptosis. The triple-combination therapy successfully reversed the immunosuppressive tumor stroma toward the immunostimulatory microenvironment (Fig. 6.2) [5].

These results also suggest that the SDF1α/CXCR4 pathway can directly mediate transition to an EMT phenotype in HCC cells in a hypoxic microenvironment. Collectively, these data may explain the unaltered progression of the disease at distant sites in the face of sorafenib treatment. Indeed, CXCR4 blockade prevented EMT despite persistent hypoxia, reduced metastatic burden, and increased survival in mice with HCC. These findings may be relevant not only for sorafenib but also for any other hypoxia-inducing therapy in HCC.

Furthermore, in addition to $Gr\text{-}1^+$ myeloid cells, as stated above, there is an increase in M2-type TAMs and Tregs in HCA-1 tumors after sorafenib treatment, indicating the induction of an immunosuppressive microenvironment in sorafenib-treated HCCs. In these HCCs CXCR4 blockade reduced the infiltration of these

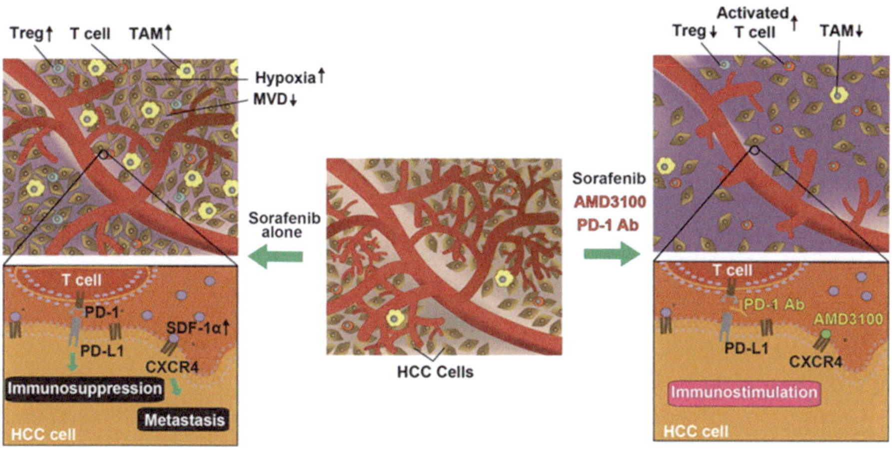

Fig. 6.2 Combination therapeutic strategy modulating the immunosuppressive microenvironment for cancer treatment. Increased intratumoral hypoxia after sorafenib treatment–caused by reduced microvascular density (MVD)–increased expression of PD-L1 and SDF-1α, and the recruitment of immunosuppressive bone marrow-derived cells (BMDCs) and regulatory T cells (Tregs) in hepatocellular carcinoma (HCC). These effects were prevented when combining sorafenib with AMD3100, a CXCR4 antagonist, which facilitated immunotherapy with anti-PD-1 antibodies

immunosuppressive cells despite persistent hypoxia but failed to promote antitumor cellular immune responses. Therefore, ICB using anti-PD-1 antibodies was added to CXCR4 blockade and sorafenib treatment, and this treatment was safe and could facilitate antitumor immune responses by increasing the infiltration and activation of $CD8^+$ T lymphocytes inside the tumor. The triple combination treatment inhibited both the growth of the primary tumor and the formation of lung metastases in orthotopic murine HCCs and regressed established tumors in a genetically engineered mouse model of HCC in mice with underlying liver cirrhosis. These data from preclinical study highlights that the clinical relevance of studying the role of the immune microenvironment in resistance to antiangiogenic treatment as well as for the future development of immunotherapy in HCC.

Unfortunately, testing triple combination therapies is challenging in clinical setting for several reasons. Hand-foot syndrome occurs most frequently by sorafenib and it is important to control this adverse event to continue this therapy. Furthermore, diarrhea, appetite loss, and fatigue are also well known effect of sorafenib. Nivolumab, anti-PD-1 antibody, is known to have some severe adverse effect, such as interstitial pneumonia, myasthenia gravis, thyroid deficiency, type I diabetes, and more. Although this triple combination therapy may potentially be a more effective treatment for immunotherapy in HCC, further investigation is needed to overcome the adverse event from these drugs to use this treatment safely in clinical setting.

6.11 Future Perspectives

Immunotherapy using ICBs has already shown unprecedented efficacy in intractable cancers such as advanced melanoma and lung cancer. This approach is currently in clinical testing in advanced HCC patients. The evidence from pre-clinical studies in animal models further support the development of PD-L1/PD-1 inhibitors in this disease.

Therapy with ICBs is most likely to succeed in combination with other surgical, cytotoxic, immune or targeted therapies. Combination of ICBs with local ablative therapies such as RFA or cryoablation – which may induce tumor antigen release/damage associated molecular patters (DAMPs) – would particularly promising approaches. However, optimal integration of ICBs with systemic treatments (e.g., sorafenib, lenvatinib, regorafenib) will require further mechanistic understanding of treatment interactions.

Our group has been pursuing such mechanistic studies in preclinical models. For example, our recent reports indicated an important role for the dose of anti-angiogenic therapy used. In a mouse model of breast cancer, administration of anti-mouse VEGFR2 neutralizing antibody (DC101) at a low dose (10 mg/kg) normalized the structure and function of the tumor vasculature, and promoted anti-tumor immunity. Interestingly, the tumor-associated macrophage population showed a reduction in the M2 (pro-tumor) phenotype. Treg activity was also reduced in the low-dose DC101 group. In contrast, when administered in higher doses (40 mg/kg), DC101 treatment induced vascular pruning, increased tissue hypoxia within the tumor, and increased M2-type macrophages and Tregs. These experiments suggest a potentially beneficial effect of titration of anti-VEGFR2 therapy on the immune response in tumors. However, recent data also showed that ICBs could affect the vascular structure and function. This introduces another layer of complexity in the interaction between antiangiogenics and ICBs. Whether combining anti-PD-1 antibodies with anti-VEGFR2 antibodies or with multi-targeted TKIs (regorafenib, lenvatinib) will enhance anti-tumor immunity in HCC and what dose/schedule regimens will achieve this remains currently unknown.

Finally, the integration of ICBs – especially when used in combination with other agents – will have to address the safety concerns specific to this population of patients such as hepatotoxicity. The potential risk of fueling acute exacerbation of viral hepatitis in HBV/HCV positive patients will need to be elucidated and the carefully be observed in the clinical setting.

Addressing these issues will greatly help the field bring to fruition the great promise of these novel immunotherapeutics in this intractable disease.

Conflicts of Interest DGD receives research funding from Merrimack, Leap Tx, Bristol-Meyers-Squibb and Bayer.

Funding DGD's work is supported through NIH grants P01-CA080124, R01-CA159258, R21-CA139168 and Proton Beam/Federal Share Program, and the American Cancer Society grant 120733-RSG-11- 073-01-TBG.

References

1. Killock D. Liver cancer: regorafenib – a new RESORCE in HCC. Nat Rev Clin Oncol. 2017;14:70–1.
2. Ignacio M, Bruno S, Cheung YT, Chiun H, Masatoshi KSCT, et al. Nivolumab dose escalation and expansion in patients with advanced hepatocellular carcinoma (HCC): the CheckMate 040 study. 2017 Gastrointestinal Cancers Symposium 2017.
3. Chen Y, Ramjiawan RR, Reiberger T, Ng MR, Hato T, Huang Y, et al. CXCR4 inhibition in tumor microenvironment facilitates anti-programmed death receptor-1 immunotherapy in sorafenib-treated hepatocellular carcinoma in mice. Hepatology. 2015;61:1591–602.
4. Chen Y, Huang Y, Reiberger T, Duyverman AM, Huang P, Samuel R, et al. Differential effects of sorafenib on liver versus tumor fibrosis mediated by stromal-derived factor 1 alpha/C-X-C receptor type 4 axis and myeloid differentiation antigen-positive myeloid cell infiltration in mice. Hepatology. 2014;59:1435–47.
5. Chen Y, Duda DG. Targeting immunosuppression after standard sorafenib treatment to facilitate immune checkpoint blockade in hepatocellular carcinoma – an auto-commentary on clinical potential and future development. Oncoimmunology. 2015;4:e1029703.
6. Llovet JM, Ricci S, Mazzaferro V, Hilgard P, Gane E, Blanc JF, et al. Sorafenib in advanced hepatocellular carcinoma. N Engl J Med. 2008;359:378–90.
7. Cheng AL, Kang YK, Chen Z, Tsao CJ, Qin S, Kim JS, et al. Efficacy and safety of sorafenib in patients in the Asia-Pacific region with advanced hepatocellular carcinoma: a phase III randomised, double-blind, placebo-controlled trial. Lancet Oncol. 2009;10:25–34.
8. Zhu AX, Rosmorduc O, Evans TR, Ross PJ, Santoro A, Carrilho FJ, et al. SEARCH: a phase III, randomized, double-blind, placebo-controlled trial of sorafenib plus erlotinib in patients with advanced hepatocellular carcinoma. J Clin Oncol. 2015;33:559–66.
9. Lencioni R, Llovet JM, Han G, Tak WY, Yang J, Guglielmi A, et al. Sorafenib or placebo plus TACE with doxorubicin-eluting beads for intermediate stage HCC: the SPACE trial. J Hepatol. 2016;64:1090–8.
10. Moriguchi M, Umemura A, Itoh Y. Current status and future prospects of chemotherapy for advanced hepatocellular carcinoma. Clin J Gastroenterol. 2016;9:184–90.
11. Cheng AL, Kang YK, Lin DY, Park JW, Kudo M, Qin S, et al. Sunitinib versus sorafenib in advanced hepatocellular cancer: results of a randomized phase III trial. J Clin Oncol. 2013;31:4067–75.
12. Zhu AX, Kudo M, Assenat E, Cattan S, Kang YK, Lim HY, et al. Effect of everolimus on survival in advanced hepatocellular carcinoma after failure of sorafenib: the EVOLVE-1 randomized clinical trial. JAMA. 2014;312:57–67.
13. Zhu AX, Baron AD, Malfertheiner P, Kudo M, Kawazoe S, Pezet D, et al. Ramucirumab as second-line treatment in patients with advanced hepatocellular carcinoma: analysis of REACH trial results by child-pugh score. JAMA Oncol. 2016.
14. Hubbard S. Exelixis announces outcome from analysis of the phase 3 CELESTIAL trial of cabozantinib in patients with advanced hepatocellular carcinoma. 2016.

15. Finn RS, Kang YK, Mulcahy M, Polite BN, Lim HY, Walters I, et al. Phase II, open-label study of brivanib as second-line therapy in patients with advanced hepatocellular carcinoma. Clin Cancer Res. 2012;18:2090–8.
16. Johnson PJ, Qin S, Park JW, Poon RT, Raoul JL, Philip PA, et al. Brivanib versus sorafenib as first-line therapy in patients with unresectable, advanced hepatocellular carcinoma: results from the randomized phase III BRISK-FL study. J Clin Oncol. 2013;31:3517–24.
17. Llovet JM, Decaens T, Raoul JL, Boucher E, Kudo M, Chang C, et al. Brivanib in patients with advanced hepatocellular carcinoma who were intolerant to sorafenib or for whom sorafenib failed: results from the randomized phase III BRISK-PS study. J Clin Oncol. 2013;31:3509–16.
18. Cainap C, Qin S, Huang WT, Chung IJ, Pan H, Cheng Y, et al. Linifanib versus Sorafenib in patients with advanced hepatocellular carcinoma: results of a randomized phase III trial. J Clin Oncol. 2015;33:172–9.
19. Rimassa L, Abbadessa G, Personeni N, Porta C, Borbath I, Daniele B, et al. Tumor and circulating biomarkers in patients with second-line hepatocellular carcinoma from the randomized phase II study with tivantinib. Oncotarget. 2016;7:72622–33.
20. Pievsky D, Pyrsopoulos N. Profile of tivantinib and its potential in the treatment of hepatocellular carcinoma: the evidence to date. J Hepatocell Carcinoma. 2016;3:69–76.
21. Ikeda M, Okusaka T, Mitsunaga S, Ueno H, Tamai T, Suzuki T, et al. Safety and pharmacokinetics of lenvatinib in patients with advanced hepatocellular carcinoma. Clin Cancer Res. 2016;22:1385–94.
22. Ikeda K, Kudo M, Kawazoe S, Osaki Y, Ikeda M, Okusaka T, et al. Phase 2 study of lenvatinib in patients with advanced hepatocellular carcinoma. J Gastroenterol. 2016.
23. Eisai Co. L. PHASE III trial of anticancer agent lenvima® as first-line treatment for unresectable hepatocellular carcinoma meets primary endpoint. 2017.
24. Hiratsuka S, Duda DG, Huang Y, Goel S, Sugiyama T, Nagasawa T, et al. C-X-C receptor type 4 promotes metastasis by activating p38 mitogen-activated protein kinase in myeloid differentiation antigen (Gr-1)-positive cells. Proc Natl Acad Sci U S A. 2011;108:302–7.
25. El-Serag HB. Hepatocellular carcinoma. N Engl J Med. 2011;365:1118–27.
26. Greten TF, Duffy AG, Korangy F. Hepatocellular carcinoma from an immunologic perspective. Clin Cancer Res. 2013;19:6678–85.
27. Nakamoto N, Cho H, Shaked A, Olthoff K, Valiga ME, Kaminski M, et al. Synergistic reversal of intrahepatic HCV-specific CD8 T cell exhaustion by combined PD-1/CTLA-4 blockade. PLoS Pathog. 2009;5:e1000313.
28. Golden-Mason L, Palmer BE, Kassam N, Townshend-Bulson L, Livingston S, McMahon BJ, et al. Negative immune regulator Tim-3 is overexpressed on T cells in hepatitis C virus infection and its blockade rescues dysfunctional CD4+ and CD8+ T cells. J Virol. 2009;83:9122–30.
29. Schurich A, Khanna P, Lopes AR, Han KJ, Peppa D, Micco L, et al. Role of the coinhibitory receptor cytotoxic T lymphocyte antigen-4 on apoptosis-Prone CD8 T cells in persistent hepatitis B virus infection. Hepatology. 2011;53:1494–503.
30. Ormandy LA, Farber A, Cantz T, Petrykowska S, Wedemeyer H, Horning M, et al. Direct ex vivo analysis of dendritic cells in patients with hepatocellular carcinoma. World J Gastroenterol. 2006;12:3275–82.
31. Ormandy LA, Hillemann T, Wedemeyer H, Manns MP, Greten TF, Korangy F. Increased populations of regulatory T cells in peripheral blood of patients with hepatocellular carcinoma. Cancer Res. 2005;65:2457–64.
32. Hoechst B, Ormandy LA, Ballmaier M, Lehner F, Kruger C, Manns MP, et al. A new population of myeloid-derived suppressor cells in hepatocellular carcinoma patients induces CD4(+)CD25(+)Foxp3(+) T cells. Gastroenterology. 2008;135:234–43.

33. Hodi FS, O'Day SJ, McDermott DF, Weber RW, Sosman JA, Haanen JB, et al. Improved survival with ipilimumab in patients with metastatic melanoma. N Engl J Med. 2010;363:711–23.
34. Tian L, Goldstein A, Wang H, Ching Lo H, Sun Kim I, Welte T, et al. Mutual regulation of tumour vessel normalization and immunostimulatory reprogramming. Nature. 2017;544:250–4.
35. Hato T, Goyal L, Greten TF, Duda DG, Zhu AX. Immune checkpoint blockade in hepatocellular carcinoma: current progress and future directions. Hepatology. 2014;60:1776–82.

Chapter 7
Glypican-3 as a Target for Immune Based Therapy in Hepatocellular Carcinoma

Yi-Fan Zhang, Jessica Hong, and Mitchell Ho

7.1 Introduction

Glypican-3 (GPC3) is a glycerophosphatidylinositol (GPI) anchored cell surface heparan sulfate proteoglycan. GPC3 is a 70 kDa protein core with heparan sulfate modifications, that attaches to the cell surface via a glycosylphosphatidylinositol (GPI) anchor at the C terminus. GPC3 was partially furin-cleaved between Arg358 and Ser359, generating a 30-kDa C-terminal fragment and an 40-kDa N-terminal fragment [1]. All the glypicans have a conserved pattern of 14 cysteine residues, which form the intramolecular disulfide linkages that connect both N and C termini [2, 3]. Four isoforms of GPC3 cDNA can been found in the GenBank; among them, Isoform 2 of GPC3 is the most common [4]. Human and mouse GPC3 proteins share 94% sequence identity [1]. GPC3 is expressed in human embryo, fetus and placental tissues [5]. It is not expressed in normal adult tissue [6], but is overexpressed in HCC [7], hepatoblastoma [8], solid pseudopapillary neoplasm type of pancreatic cancer [9], Wilms tumor [8], malignant melanoma [10], a group of ovarian clear cell adenocarcinoma [11], Testicular germ cell tumors [12], testicular and ovarian yolk sac tumors [13], Merkel cell carcinoma [14], thyroid cancer [15] and lung squamous cell carcinoma [16]. Particularly, GPC3 is overexpressed in 79% of HCC and 11% of cirrhotic nodules [17]; HCC arising in cirrhotic liver are more likely to be GPC3 positive [17]. GPC3 expression is much higher in early HCCs than in cirrhosis, indicating that the transition from cirrhosis to early HCC is associated with a significant increase of GPC3 expression [18]. Thus, GPC3 is a suitable HCC marker and prognostic factor of HCC, and has been a target candidate in various investigational immunotherapies (Fig. 7.1).

Y.-F. Zhang • J. Hong • M. Ho (✉)
Laboratory of Molecular Biology, National Cancer Institute, Bethesda, MD 20892, USA
e-mail: homi@mail.nih.gov

T.F. Greten (ed.), *Immunotherapy of Hepatocellular Carcinoma*,
DOI 10.1007/978-3-319-64958-0_7

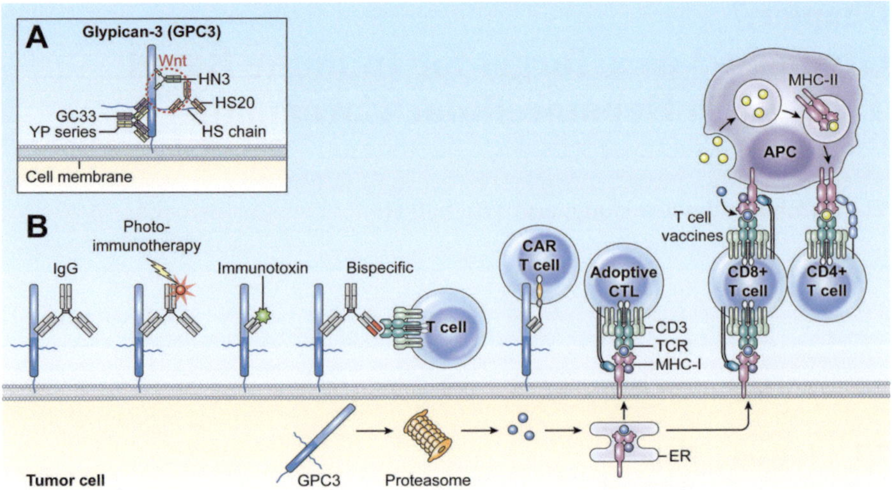

Fig. 7.1 (**a**) The epitopes of anti-GPC3 antibodies. (**b**) The therapeutic formats for anti-GPC3 immunotherapies

7.2 GPC3 Vaccinations

Cancer vaccinations have been used to prevent cancer recurrence because large tumor burden can induce immune-tolerance [19]. Therefore, a suitable tumor-specific antigen for cancer vaccine should be expressed early in cancer development, and be able to induce effective immune response. As discussed above, GPC3 is expressed early in HCC development. Interestingly, GPC3 can induce GPC3-specific cytotoxic T lymphocytes (CTLs) in HCC patients treated with radiofrequency ablation or trans-catheter arterial chemo-embolization (TACE), but not surgical resection [20]. It was also observed that autologous formalin-fixed tumor vaccine after TACE and radiofrequency ablation (RFA) lowered the recurrence risk, and induce GPC3-specific CTLs in peripheral blood [21]. Therefore, GPC3 vaccines have been developed for the treatment of liver cancer.

Compared to tissue, protein, and DNA immunization [22], peptide vaccines can be directly taken up by the antigen-presenting cells. This is because peptide vaccines can directly bind the specific HLA in the patients and bypass antigen-processing in the host. Thus peptide vaccines can be engineered to preferentially induce CD8+ or CD4+ T cells, which may require optimization [23]. Short peptides (8 amino acids) are presented very efficiently by dendritic cells. Long peptides (15–35 amino acids) are presented less efficiently, but still much more efficiently presented than proteins, by dendritic cells (not B or T cells) [24, 25].

MHC class I restricted peptides are designed to elicit CD8+ CTLs response. From the group of peptides conserved between human and mouse, the HLA-A*24:02-restricted $GPC3_{298-306}$ peptide (EYILSLEEL) was selected because it is predicted in silico to bind both human HLA-A24 and mouse K^d. Furthermore, it induced mouse CTL by vaccination [26]. From the group of conserved peptides, the HLA-A2-restricted $GPC3_{144–152}$ peptide (FVGEFFTDV) was selected because it is predicted in silico to bind human HLA-A2, and the dendritic cells pulsed with the peptide activated CTL in HLA-A2.1 (HHD) transgenic mice [27]. Both A24-$GPC3_{298–306}$ and A2-$GPC3_{144–152}$ peptides activated CTLs from patient's peripheral blood mononuclear cells (PBMCs) [27]. In a recent Phase II study with HCC patients after curative surgery [28], the $GPC3_{298–306}$ peptide was given to HLA-A24-positive patients, and the $GPC3_{144–152}$ peptide was given to HLA-A2-positive patients. GPC3 peptides were emulsified with incomplete Freund's adjuvant and injected intradermally. The first vaccine was given within 4 weeks after curative surgery, followed by one injection every 2 weeks for five times and then one injection every 2 months for four times. The GPC3 targeting CTLs can be detected in 35 of the 41 patients (85.4%) after vaccination. Of the patients bearing GPC3+ HCC, vaccination lowered the 1-year recurrence rate from 48% to 24%. During the second year, when the vaccination was discontinued, the recurrence rate of vaccinated patients (52.4%) was closer to that of the non-vaccinated patients (61.9%), suggesting a loss of memory. Many recurrent patients still have GPC3 specific CTLs, suggesting that such CTLs are not enough at the time of recurrence. CTLs isolated from needle-biopsy specimens of one recurrent tumor expressed more PD-1 than the CD8+ T cells in PBMCs, suggesting the induction of anergy. Two recurrent patients having higher number of GPC3 specific CTLs lack GPC3 expression in the recurrent tumor, suggesting that vaccines towards other tumor antigens might be needed to protect such patients from recurrence. In a study conducted by Sawada et al. (2012), an autopsy was done on a HCC patient after ongoing GPC3 peptide vaccination [29]. The immunological analysis and autopsy showed that after the second vaccination, the number of GPC3 peptide-specific CTLs increased from 0 to 84 which could correlate with GPC3 peptide vaccine response since it showed an increased number of CTLs. Prior to vaccination, a liver biopsy was taken which revealed well-differentiated HCC. Immunohistochemical staining showed that prior to vaccination, GPC3 and HLA class I was found in the cytoplasm and membranes of HCC cells along with a few CD8 positive T cells in the tissues. An autopsy was done 2 h following death and found multiple nodular lesions with central necrosis in the right lobe of the liver. Immunohistochemical staining showed GPC3 positive carcinoma cells with an infiltration of CD8 positive T cells in carcinoma but not within cirrhotic areas. The cause of death was not likely to be due to vaccine-induced liver injury. CD68 positive macrophages were found around the necrotic area of cirrhotic nodules as well as CD8 positive cells which suggest that the carcinoma cells were attacked by CD8 positive T cells that could lead to necrosis. In addition, 3 of 33 patients that received GPC3 peptide vaccination in a phase I trial showed tumor necrosis on CT scans. Overall, GPC3 peptide vaccination targeting CD8+ T cells has limited efficacy and needs further improvement.

Interestingly, the MHC class I restricted A2-$GPC3_{144–152}$ peptide and A24 $GPC3_{298–306}$ peptide induced CD4+ T cell response in roughly 2/3 of patients, who have prolonged 3-year and 5-year survival, with 10/11 patients (compared to

0/5 CD4+ T cell response-negative patients) alive after 5 years. More strikingly, even without GPC3 specific CD8+ T cells, the patients with the CD4+ T cell response had prolonged 3-year and 5-year survival, with 5/5 patients (compared to 0/3 CD4+ T cell response negative/CD8+ T cell response negative patients) alive after 5 years [30]. Although it is unclear whether CD4+ T cell response is the cause or the consequence of cytotoxicity, it is consistent with the previous observation that stimulation of CD4+ T cells alone can mediate tumor regression [31] and CD4+ T cells are required to maintain long-term immunologic memory [32]. A recent study showed that CD4+ T cells were indeed involved in HCC tumorigenesis, as they were lost in non-alcoholic fatty liver disease and their depletion accelerated HCC carcinogenesis. Therefore, CD4+ T cells may play an important role in HCC therapy [33]. These studies may suggest that GPC3 vaccines targeting CD4+ T cells may be promising.

A short peptide derived from human adenovirus type 5 E1A, induced specific T cell tolerance [34, 35] which can be converted to anti-tumor response when presented on dendritic cells [36]. This is probably because it can skip the antigen-process step in dendritic cells and directly bind MHC-I molecules on target cells in vivo. This is peptide specific, as the dendritic cell pulsed with another peptide vaccine (a p53:264–272 peptide vaccine) in vitro did not show significant advantage over direct peptide based vaccination in patient response or survival [37]. The clinical trial result with GPC3 short peptides showed the expression of PD-1 in one of the recurrent patients, and the lack of long-term protection suggest some immune tolerance. To avoid such cases, long-peptides, which are processed in DC, can be designed. Peptides of 23 residues or greater are also required to stimulate a high affinity MHC-II restricted T cell response [38]. To induce CD4+ T cell response and avoid immune tolerance, the MHC class II restricted GPC3-derived long peptides have been developed [30]. $GPC3_{92–116}$ (LP1), $GPC3_{137–161}$ (LP2), $GPC3_{289–313}$ (LP3), $GPC3_{386–412}$ (LP4), and $GPC3_{556–576}$ (LP5) were predicted to bind multiple frequently observed HLA class II molecules (encoded by DPB1*05:01, DRB1*07:01, DRB1*08:03, DRB1*09:01, DRB1*13:02, or DRB1*15:02 alleles) with overlapping high-consensus percentile ranks. They bound antigen-presenting cells (APC) and induced peptide-specific CD4+ T cell responses from most healthy donors, and LP1, 2, 4, and 5 was presented by APC pulsed with recombinant GPC3. The preventative power of these peptides remains to be tested in patients.

The formula of peptide vaccines can also be optimized to greatly improve the balance between CTL immunity versus tolerance [39]. Compared to the incomplete Freund's adjuvant emulsified peptides, liposome-coupled GPC3-derived epitope peptide induced stronger CTL response at the same or lower doses [40]. Two vaccinations of liposome coupled GPC3 peptide A2-$GPC3_{144–152}$ before tumor inoculation, along with one vaccination after tumor inoculation, inhibited the growth of GPC3+ xenograft tumors. Its effect on long-term immune memory and the preventative power in patients remains to be tested.

7.3 GPC3 Antibody Therapeutics

Antibody-based therapies are being developed for the treatment of liver cancer. Antibodies can be engineered into various clinical formats. The therapeutic effect of antibody-related therapies is based on the biological function of the binding and the effector function linked to the binding domain, which we will discuss in detail as follows.

7.3.1 Generation of Anti-GPC3 Antibodies

To avoid excessive immune tolerance due to sequence homology in mice, Nakano et al. immunized MRL/lpr (Fas-deficient) mice, which develop an autoimmune syndrome that is associated with excessive production of autoantibodies. The research team immunized with soluble GPC3, lacking the GPI-anchoring domain, and isolated three antibodies recognizing N-fragment and four antibodies recognizing C-fragment. They further found the antibodies recognizing C-fragment have stronger antibody-dependent cell mediated cytotoxicity (ADCC) and complement dependent cytotoxicity (CDC). Therefore, they used GPC3 C-fragment as the immunogen for MRL/lpr mice and selected antibody GC33 for its strongest binding [1]. Our group at the U.S. National Cancer Institute generates a group of high affinity antibodies (YP7, YP8, YP9 and YP9.1) through high-throughput flow cytometry subtractive screening on GPC3+ and GPC3- cells [41]. We immunized BALB/c mice with a 50-mer peptide (residues 511–560) corresponding to the C-terminal end of cell-surface GPC3. It is the consensus sequence among the four different splice variants of GPC3 [4], The mouse YP7, YP8 and YP9.1 antibodies have been humanized recently for clinical applications [42]. We also screened a human antibody single domain VH library against recombinant GPC3 protein by phage display technology and isolated HN3, which recognizes a highly conformational epitope that requires both N- and C-fragments of GPC3 but does not need the heparan sulfate chains [43]. The HN3 recognize a distinct epitope from YP7 and GC33 and has unique functional properties that can inhibit Wnt/Yap signaling in liver cancer cells [43] [44]. We then panned a human scFv phage library against GPC3 protein and isolated HS20, which recognizes the heparan sulfate chains of GPC3 [45]. The HS20 human antibody binding requires a particular structure with the sulfation of both the C2 position (2-O-sulfation) and C6 position (6-O-sulfation) [46]. The binding epitopes of these antibodies are shown schematically in Fig. 7.1a.

Depending on the cell context, GPC3 can either inhibit or promote cell proliferation. During embryonic development, GPC3 prevents overgrowth as the GPC3 deletion mutations are associated with Simpson-Golabi-Behmel syndrome characterized by macrosomia [47]. In HCC, however, all the data show that GPC3 promotes tumor growth: GPC3 silencing inhibits cell growth [48], and extracellular soluble GPC3 can function as a dominant negative form to inhibit cell growth [49]. The growth effect of GPC3 in HCC cells is related to Wnt signaling, which is abnormal in 95% of HCC patients [50]. GPC3 binds both Wnt [51] and its receptor Frizzled [52]. The HN3 single domain antibody inhibits Wnt signaling [44] and HCC growth [43]. Similarly, HS20 blocks Wnt-binding site on the heparan sulfate chains of GPC3 [46] and inhibits exogenous Wnt-induced cell growth [45]. Besides cell proliferation, GPC3 is also involved in HCC cell migration and motility [53]. GPC3 knockdown inhibits cell motility and migration. This is partly due to the interaction between GPC3 heparan sulfate chain and hepatocyte growth factor (HGF). The HS20 human antibody inhibits HGF-mediated HCC cell migration and motility [53]. GPC3 has also been reported to interact with Fibroblast growth factor (FGF) [54], Insulin-like growth factor (IGF)-II and IGF-1R [55], Hedgehog [56], Glucose transporter 1 (Glut1) [57], Glucose transporter 4 (Glut4) [58], and Low density lipoprotein receptor-related protein 1 (LRP1) [59]. The GPC3 furin cleavage downregulates the sulfation of the heparan sulfate chain, and switches the hedgehog binding site from the heparan sulfate chain to the core protein, and switches from competing with Patched to facilitating Patched for the hedgehog binding [60]. It remains interesting to see the role of these signaling interactions in HCC tumorigenesis using new anti-GPC3 antibodies and test their therapeutic effects.

Ishiguro et al. used the anti-glypican 3 antibody as an antitumor agent against human liver cancer [61]. The mAb GC33 was found to inhibit growth of Huh-7 and caused tumor remission in HepG2. In addition, mice treated with 5 mg/kg GC33 sustained their body weight by HepG2 xenografts, whereas the control mice had decreased body weight as the tumor progressed. The degree of tumor inhibition correlates with the level of GPC3 protein since it inhibited more in the high GPC3 SK-03 and inhibited the least in the low GPC3 Huh-7. In orthotopic tumors, after the injection of HepG2, alpha fetal protein (AFP) levels were between 10 and 100 ng/ml. When given GC33, AFP levels were <1 ng/ml, whereas mice without GC33 had increased AFP levels. After 35 days, there were no tumors observed in mice with GC33, but multiple tumors in control mice. This suggests that GC33 is effective against HepG2 in mice. Interestingly, when GC33 is combined with sorafenib, tumor inhibition is more significant compared to treating with sorafenib or GC33 alone. GC33 also maintained body weight due to weight loss due to sorafenib. By combining GC33 with a chemotherapeutic agent, the effects can be increased. Furthermore, GC33 induces ADCC in GPC3 positive hepatoma cells and can inhibit tumor growth in human liver cancer xenograft models.

The antibodies for cancer therapy are usually made in IgG1 isotype, which can induce ADCC and CDC [62]. The binding epitope, binding affinity, and target expression level affect ADCC and CDC. The GC33 [1] and humanized YP7 (hYP7) [42] antibodies can induce ADCC and modest CDC in vitro; GC33 inhibit xenograft tumor growth in vivo via macrophage-dependent ADCC [63]. In addition to ADCC and CDC, it has been shown that Wnt blocking antibodies HN3 [43, 45] and HS20 [45] inhibited xenograft tumor growth more effectively than hYP7, suggesting that inhibition of GPC3 signaling contribute to the better efficacy in vivo.

The GC33 antibody was well tolerated in the phase 1 clinical trials [64, 65]. However, in a randomized phase 2 trial, when given 1600 mg Q2W after two weekly doses no clinical benefits were shown [66], suggesting that antibodies alone may have low toxicity and modest therapeutic effects in HCC patients. Armed antibody therapeutics should be explored for better efficacy.

7.3.2 Photoimmunotherapy (PIT)

Photoimmunetherapy (PIT) [67] utilizes a monoclonal antibody conjugated to a hydrophilic photosensitizing phthalocyanine dye IRDye700DX® (IR700) to target cancer cells via exposure to near-infrared (NIR) light. PIT induces a rapid cell necrosis based on membrane disruption caused by a combination of photoinduced ligand exchange and reactive oxygen species (ROS). The antibody–photo-sensitizer conjugate is only active when it is bound to the target cell membrane. The PIT caused an increase in the blood flow and permeability of tumor vessels, permitting the delivery of relatively high concentrations of nanosized-drugs. Anti-GPC3 antibodies YP7-IR700 conjugate were given at 100 ug/mice i.v. With three exposures of NIR light on three consecutive days, 50 J/cm^2, 100 J/cm^2 and 100 J/cm^2, respectively, PIT treated mice showed significant tumor growth inhibition when exposed to the NIR light on three consecutive days compared to control mice. When only given a single exposure to PIT, no significant effect was shown. However, when given 7.5 mg of nab-paclitaxel the tumor inhibition increased. Compared to the control group, tumor inhibition was shown when treated with either nab-paclitaxel alone or nab-paclitaxel with PIT. However, tumor inhibition was significantly greater with the combination of PIT and nab-paclitaxel. Therefore, the combination of YP7-IR700 and nab-paclitaxel was more effective than the single drug alone [67]. In addition, mice that were acutely PIT treated showed a rapid accumulation of IR800-nab-paclitaxel and the tumor became clearly visible within 1 h of injection with target-to-background ratio of IR800 fluorescence [67]. Those mice that were not treated with PIT showed less IR800-nab-paclitaxel after 1 h. In addition, PIT treated mice had greater tumor fluorescence intensity by IR800-nab-paclitaxel than the control tumors. This indicates The PIT with YP7-IR700 increased the leakage of nanosized IR800-nab-paclitaxel into the tumor bed which leads to better drug efficacy. The single domain antibody HN3 was also conjugated to IR700 for PIT. Compared to YP7-IR700, HN3-IR700 accumulated similarly into tumor but achieved more homogenous intratumoral distribution. The therapeutic effect of YP7-IR700 and HN3-IR700 was similar. Given the same amount of molecules and NIR light, they both inhibit 40% tumor growth [68].

7.3.3 Immunotoxin Therapy

The pseudomonas exotoxin [69] can kill the cells by inhibiting protein synthesis after cell binding and internalizations. The native toxin can be divided into three domains: the domain I is involved in cell binding and can be replace with antibody

Fv, the function of domain II remains elusive, and the domain III inhibits protein synthesis. To construct immunotoxins using a fragment (PE38) containing domains II and III, the native binding domain (domain I) is replaced with the antibody fragment [69]. BL22, the anti-CD22/PE38 fusion protein, produced complete remission in relapsed/refractory hairy cell leukemia [70]. SS1P, the anti-mesothelin PE38, when used together with immunosuppressant pentostatin and cyclophosphamide regressed mesotheliomas in some patients [71]. Thus, the immunotoxin is a viable clinical format to treat cancer.

Anti-GPC3 immunotoxins have been generated initially in the format of Fv-PE38 fusion protein. The Wnt inhibiting HN3-PE38 regressed the HCC xenograft tumor in mice at 0.6 mg/kg, indicating that the immunotoxin format is much more effective than the naked antibody. The work has established GPC3 as a new target for immunotoxin treatment. Interestingly, not every anti-GPC3 antibody is effective in the format of an immunotoxin. The HN3-PE38 immunotoxin was much more effective and better tolerated than the YP7-PE38, indicating dual inhibition of Wnt signaling and protein synthesis is much more effective than the toxin-mediated inhibition [44].

As pointed out in a recent review [72], the immunotoxin clinical trials show that 2–5 cycles of treatment are required to obtain major clinical response that includes complete remissions [73]. However, the pseudomonas exotoxin part of the immunotoxin induces neutralizing antibodies in the majority of patients with normal immune systems, which prevent additional treatment cycles. To solve this problem, immunosuppressants can delay the formation of neutralizing antibodies and enable the patients to receive more cycles of immunotoxin treatment, thus achieve better therapeutic effects [74–78]. Directly injecting the immunotoxin into the compartmentalized tumor also helps to overcome the immunogenicity [79–81]. TACE technology is available for HCC treatment [82], and its effect on the immunogenicity of immunotoxins will need to be determined. Meanwhile, T-cell and B-cell epitopes are identified and removed in newer versions of immunotoxins [83–91]. The maximum tolerable dose of anti-GPC3 immunotoxin HN3-PE38 is 0.8 mg/kg. To increase the dose, based on previous works on immunotoxin engineering [87], the domain II of pseudomonas exotoxin, which cause non-specific cytotoxicity, was removed from the HN3-based immunotoxin; in addition, seven point mutations was made in domain III to remove the human B-cell epitopes. The resulting HN3-mPE24 has the maximum tolerable dose at 7 mg/kg, ninefolds higher than the HN3-PE38. When injected every other day for ten injections, 5 mg/kg HN3-mPE24 regressed the tumor and kept 25% of mice alive for more than 100 days, whereas 0.6 mg/kg HN3-PE38 did not. Even though the HN3-mPE24 had similar in vitro cytotoxicity and lower in vivo efficacy than HN3-PE38 at the same dose, the higher tolerable dose and lower immunogenicity of mPE24 overwhelmingly outweighed the slight loss of activity [92]. It would be interesting to further engineer the HN3-based immunotoxins by removing both B and T cell epitopes to select the best molecule for the clinical trial.

7.3.4 Bispecific Antibody

The GC33 antibody has been made into a bispecific antibody with an anti-CD3 antibody. It is a fully humanized IgG4 bispecific antibody, with a mutation to silence FcγR. Preclinical data showed that this antibody was active against GPC3-positive tumors and that corticosteroids reduced cytokine release and widened the therapeutic window. It is currently being tested in a phase I clinical trial [93].

7.3.5 Chimeric Antigen Receptor-T Cell Therapy

Chimeric antigen receptors (CAR) are antibody Fv linked via an extracellular hinge and transmembrane domain to the intracellular signaling domains of T cell receptor CD3ζ. T cells from patients are isolated, activated, genetically modified to express CAR, and infused into the patients [94]. Upon binding the antigen on the target cells, independent of MHC, the adjacent CAR will align and activate CD3ζ, and in turn activate T cells.

To enhance and sustain the T cell activation signal, the second generation CARs have included the signaling domain of co-stimulatory receptors, such as CD28 and 4-1BB, before the signaling domains of CD3ζ, to generate 28Z and BBZ CARs, respectively. The second generation anti-CD19 CAR with either CD28 or 4-1BB exhibited 79–90% complete response rates in clinical trials [94]. An anti-CD19 BBZ CAR-T expanded >1000-fold in vivo, each cell eradicating 1000 tumor cells in vivo, and a portion of these cells persisted as memory CAR+ T cells and retained anti-CD19 effector functionality [95]. Various evidence showed that CD28 induces early activation, whereas 4-1BB promotes sustained activation [96]. To further activate the T cells, the third generation CAR include two co-stimulatory domains, such as CD28, 4-1BB and OX40 (CD134), which is more similar to 4-1BB [96]. The CD28/4-1BB/CD3ζ (28BBZ) CAR T cells, targeting mesothelin, had a larger cell number in the peripheral blood 20 days after last infusion than the second generation 28Z or BBZ CAR T cells. The third generation CAR T cells had more potent antitumor effect than BBZ CAR T cells in vivo [97]. The 28BBZ CAR T cells targeting prostate-specific membrane antigen (PSMA) also showed more potent antitumor effect than the second generation CARs, and the effect of CD28 and 4-1BB appears to be additive [98]. The 28BBZ third generation CAR versus 28Z second generation CAR is being compared in a phase 1 clinical trial (NCT01853631) to treat refractory/relapsed indolent and aggressive B-cell non-Hodgkin lymphomas (NHL), targeting CD19.

The anti-GPC3 antibody GC33 was recently engineered into a third generation 28BBZ CAR with CD8 hinge, CD28 transmembrane domain and intracellular signaling domain, 4-1BB intracellular signaling domain, and CD3ζ intracellular signaling domain. Single i.v. infusion of 8 x 10^6 CAR T cells regressed subcutaneous Huh7 tumor from around 250 mm^3 to below 50 mm^3. Similar results was seen in an orthotopic Huh7 HCC model, in which the GC33 CAR T treated mice achieved 100% survival 60 days after tumor inoculation, whereas control mice all died within 45 days [99]. One week after infusion, the peripheral CAR T cell count in the subcutaneous tumor model was >350/μl, compared to <100/ul irrelevent control CAR T, indicating target-induced CAR-T cell expansion. The GC33 28BBZ CAR-T is being tested in a clinical trial to treat HCC patients (NCT02395250). Besides HCC, it also regressed a lung squamous cell carcinoma xenograft in NSG mice [100]. These preclinical reports support that GPC3 is a promising target for CAR T therapy.

When induced with HCC cells in vitro, the second generation BBZ CAR preferentially produce Th-1 cytokines IFNγ and GM-CSF, 28Z preferentially produce Th-2 cytokines IL4 and IL10, and third generation 28BBZ CAR produce all the four cytokines [101]. This is different from the anti-mesothelin CAR T cells, which were cultured using another method, and secreted low or undetectable amounts of IL4, IL5, IL10 and IL17 when induced in vitro [97]. The GC33 28BBZ CAR showed the similar antitumor effect as the BBZ CAR, in NSG mice which is also deficient in B cell development [101]. Furthermore, GPC3-positive tumor xenografts can be eliminated by GPC3-CAR T cells in vivo. NSG mice were injected intraperitoneally with 2×10^6 Huh-7Ffluc cells followed by IV injection of 1×10^7 Gz, G28z, GBBz, or G28BBz T cells. Mice injected with G28z, GBBz, and G28BBz T cells had greater tumor reduction compared to the control mice. GPC3-CARs with 4-1BB endodomains have proliferative potential. They can also be used use in immunotherapy in vivo and have shown that GPC3-CAR with G28z or G28BBz have potential for therapeutic activity.

In another study, Li et al. compared CARs encoded with CD3 (Gz), as well as costimulatory domains such as CD28 (G28z), 4-1BB (GBBz), or both CD28 and 41-BB (G28BBz) [102]. GPC3-CARs can be stably expressed on T cells, with their cell surface expressing a median of 79.2% for Gz, 80% for both G28z and GBBz, and 70% for G28BBz. Altogether, it generated CAR T-cell lines containing 95% CD3 positive T cells composing of CD4 and CD8 positive T cells. GPC3 CAR T cells recognize and kill GPC3-positive tumor cells such as HepG2, Huh-7, Hep3B, G401, and A549 that was modified to express GPC3. It did not target the unmodified A549 cells or the negative controls such as GD2 specific CAR T cells, confirming that the CARs were specific to targeting GPC3-positive tumor cells.

The HN3 single domain antibody has been engineered into a 4th generation CAR T with CD28, CD27 and 41BB costimulatory domains, a CD3ζ signaling domain fused to a FKBP-iCasp9 apoptosis inducing gene, and showed strong in vitro cytotoxicity towards HCC cells. Sorafenib priming (24 h, IC10 concentration) prior to CAR T incubation boosted the specific lysis up to 25%, suggesting combination of sorafenib and anti GPC3 CAR T can be a promising strategy [103].

7.4 Adoptive TCR Expressing-T Cells

Adoptive T cells targeting GPC3 has been explored [104]. Peptides were coimmunoprecipitated with HLA-A2 from a liver cancer cell line HepG2 cells, which is HLA-A2+ GPC3+. GPC3367 (TIHDSIQYV) and GPC3326 (FIDKKVLKV) were among the top 30% most abundant peptides, and GPC3367 were predicted with higher affinity. Monocyte-derived dendritic cells from an HLA-A2-negative donor were cotransfected with GPC3 and HLA-A2, and used to stimulate CD8+ enriched T cells from the same donor. The GPC3-specific, HLA-A2 specific, A2-GPC3367 specific, and the IFNγ -secreting cells can be isolated. The dominant TCR clone P1–1 was identified. P1–1 expressing CTL had a similar cytotoxicity as CAR-T cells when measured in vitro [104]. When P1–1 transduced CD8+ T cells were tested in vivo on established HepG2 s.c. xenograft tumors, it inhibited tumor growth initially, but only slowed down tumor growth thereafter. The lack of CTL infiltration and a reduced or mosaic pattern of GPC3 expression in the tumor was observed. CAR-T cells usually contain both CD4+ and CD8+ T cells, and as mentioned above, the CD4+ T cells may also contribute to the anti-tumor activity in liver cancer. The second and third generation CAR-T cells have costimulatory-signaling domain, which can enhance and sustain T-cell activation.

7.5 Conclusion

GPC3 is an emerging tumor target for liver cancer therapy. It is expressed early in HCC and involved in HCC tumorigenesis. The GPC3 peptide vaccines are explored to prevent HCC recurrence after surgery. GPC3 short peptide designed in silico to activate CD8+ T cells were safe and they lowered the tumor recurrence rate in HCC patients after surgery, but the protection gradually lost in the following year after vaccination stopped [28], and the patients with the best protection had anti-GPC3 CD4+ T cell response regardless of CD8+ T cell response [30]. To enhance the protective effect, the liposome coupled GPC3 peptide was more potent than the Freund's adjuvant emulsified peptide to induce CTL response in vitro [39]. The most abundantly presented GPC3 peptide by HLA-A2 was identified by coimmunoprecipitation and it can induce CTL responses in vitro, and the dominating clone P1–1 can be overexpressed in CTL to inhibit HepG2 tumor growth in mice in early phase [104]. Long peptides have been developed and validated in vitro to induce CD4+ T cell response [30].

The antibody-related therapies have been developed to treat established HCC. Anti-GPC3 antibodies GC33, YP7, HN3, HS20 has been generated by using hybridoma and phage display technologies. The GC33 and YP7 recognize the C terminus, the HN3 human single domain antibody targets a conformation epitope on the protein core of GPC3, and the HS20 human IgG binds heparan sulfate chains. The HN3 and HS20 antibodies block Wnt/Yap signaling via two distinct sites on

GPC3. HS20 also inhibits HGF signaling. The IgG-based antibodies alone and photoimmunotherapies can slow down tumor growth, whereas the HN3 immunotoxin can regress the tumor. The Wnt-blocking HN3 immunotoxin is more potent than YP7 immunotoxin. Using a re-engineered toxin, the HN3 immunotoxin can be given at a high dose repeatedly, regress HCC xenograft tumor and cause complete remission in mice. Further engineering of the HN3 immunotoxin for the removal of various human T- and B- cell epitopes is ongoing for clinical development. The CAR T-cell format also showed great promise. The GC33 CAR T cells regressed established HCC xenograft tumors in mice, and the HN3 CAR T cells are being tested in the preclinical stage. Various versions of the CAR effector parts are being evaluated and compared to improve the anti-tumor efficacy in liver cancer.

Liver cancer remains one of the most common and deadly cancers in the world. Currently there is no effective therapy. Antibody-based cancer therapies including immunotoxins, CAR T cells, cancer vaccines, and bispecific antibodies are being developed for clinical use. These ongoing preclinical and clinical studies will further define the utility of GPC3 as a target for liver cancer therapy.

Acknowledgement This research was supported by the Intramural Research Program of the NIH, National Cancer Institute, Center for Cancer Research. We would like to thank Alan Hoofring and Ethan Tyler, NIH Medical Arts Design Section, for making the figure and Douglas Joubert, NIH Library Editing Service, for editing the text.

Conflict of Interest Statement The authors declare no conflict of interest.

References

1. Nakano K, Orita T, Nezu J, Yoshino T, Ohizumi I, Sugimoto M, et al. Anti-glypican 3 antibodies cause ADCC against human hepatocellular carcinoma cells. Biochem Biophys Res Commun. 2009;378:279–84.
2. Kim M-S, Saunders AM, Hamaoka BY, Beachy PA, Leahy DJ. Structure of the protein core of the glypican dally-like and localization of a region important for hedgehog signaling. Proc Natl Acad Sci. 2011;108:13112–7.
3. Svensson G, Awad W, Håkansson M, Mani K, Logan DT. Crystal structure of N-glycosylated human glypican-1 core protein: structure of two loops evolutionarily conserved in vertebrate glypican-1. J Biol Chem. 2012;287:14040–51.
4. Ho M, Kim H. Glypican-3: a new target for cancer immunotherapy. Eur J Cancer. 2011;47:333–8.
5. Iglesias BV, Centeno G, Pascuccelli H, Ward F, Peters MG, Filmus J, et al. Expression pattern of glypican-3 (GPC3) during human embryonic and fetal development. Histol Histopathol. 2008;23:1333–40.
6. Ligato S, Mandich D, Cartun RW. Utility of glypican-3 in differentiating hepatocellular carcinoma from other primary and metastatic lesions in FNA of the liver: an immunocytochemical study. Mod Pathol. 2008;21:626–31.
7. Capurro M, Wanless IR, Sherman M, Deboer G, Shi W, Miyoshi E, et al. Glypican-3: a novel serum and histochemical marker for hepatocellular carcinoma. Gastroenterology. 2003;125:89–97.

8. Toretsky JA, Zitomersky NL, Eskenazi AE, Voigt RW, Strauch ED, Sun CC, et al. Glypican-3 expression in wilms tumor and hepatoblastoma. J Pediatr Hematol Oncol. 2001;23:496–9.
9. Hav M, De Potter A, Ferdinande L, Van Bockstal M, Lem D, Eav S, et al. Glypican-3 is a marker for solid pseudopapillary neoplasm of the pancreas. Histopathology. 2011;59:1278–9.
10. Nakatsura T, Kageshita T, Ito S, Wakamatsu K, Monji M, Ikuta Y, et al. Identification of Glypican-3 as a novel tumor marker for melanoma. Clin Cancer Res. 2004;10:6612–21.
11. Maeda D, Ota S, Takazawa Y, Aburatani H, Nakagawa S, Yano T, et al. Glypican-3 expression in clear cell adenocarcinoma of the ovary. Mod Pathol. 2009;22:824–32.
12. Zynger DL, Dimov ND, Luan C, Tean Teh B, Yang XJ. Glypican 3: a novel marker in testicular germ cell tumors. Am J Surg Pathol. 2006;30:1570–5. doi:10.1097/01.pas.0000213322.89670.48.
13. Zynger DL, McCallum JC, Luan C, Chou PM, Yang XJ. Glypican 3 has a higher sensitivity than alpha-fetoprotein for testicular and ovarian yolk sac tumour: immunohistochemical investigation with analysis of histological growth patterns. Histopathology. 2010;56:750–7.
14. He H, Fang W, Liu X, Weiss LM, Chu PG. Frequent expression of glypican-3 in merkel cell carcinoma: an immunohistochemical study of 55 cases. Appl Immunohistochem Mol Morphol. 2009;17:40–6. doi:10.1097/PAI.0b013e31817b67d1.
15. Yamanaka K, Ito Y, Okuyama N, Noda K, Matsumoto H, Yoshida H, et al. Immunohistochemical study of glypican 3 in thyroid cancer. Oncology. 2007;73:389–94.
16. Aviel-Ronen S, Lau SK, Pintilie M, Lau D, Liu N, Tsao MS, et al. Glypican-3 is overexpressed in lung squamous cell carcinoma, but not in adenocarcinoma. Mod Pathol. 2008;21:817–25.
17. Shafizadeh N, Ferrell LD, Kakar S. Utility and limitations of glypican-3 expression for the diagnosis of hepatocellular carcinoma at both ends of the differentiation spectrum. Mod Pathol. 2008;21:1011–8.
18. Libbrecht L, Severi T, Cassiman D, Borght SV, Pirenne J, Nevens F, et al. Glypican-3 expression distinguishes small hepatocellular carcinomas from cirrhosis, dysplastic nodules, and focal nodular hyperplasia-like nodules. Am J Surg Pathol. 2006;30:1405–11. doi:10.1097/01.pas.0000213323.97294.9a.
19. Gray A, Raff AB, Chiriva-Internati M, Chen S-Y, Kast WM. A paradigm shift in therapeutic vaccination of cancer patients: the need to apply therapeutic vaccination strategies in the preventive setting. Immunol Rev. 2008;222:316–27.
20. Nobuoka D, Motomura Y, Shirakawa H, Yoshikawa T, Kuronuma T, Takahashi M, et al. Radiofrequency ablation for hepatocellular carcinoma induces glypican-3 peptide-specific cytotoxic T lymphocytes. Int J Oncol. 2012;40:63–70.
21. Kawashima I, Kawashima Y, Matsuoka Y, Fujise K, Sakai H, Takahashi M, et al. Suppression of postsurgical recurrence of hepatocellular carcinoma treated with autologous formalin-fixed tumor vaccine, with special reference to glypican-3. Clin Case Rep. 2015;3:444–7.
22. Li S, Lin J, Qi C, Fu S, Xiao W, Peng B, et al. GPC3 DNA vaccine elicits potent cellular antitumor immunity against HCC in mice. Hepato-Gastroenterology. 2014;61:278–84.
23. Vreeland TJ, Hale DK, Clifton GT, Sears AK, Mittendorf EA, Peoples GE. Peptide vaccine strategies in the treatment of cancer. J Proteomics Bioinforma. 2013;6:81–4.
24. Rosalia RA, Quakkelaar ED, Redeker A, Khan S, Camps M, Drijfhout JW, et al. Dendritic cells process synthetic long peptides better than whole protein, improving antigen presentation and T-cell activation. Eur J Immunol. 2013;43:2554–65.
25. Romero P, Banchereau J, Bhardwaj N, Cockett M, Disis ML, Dranoff G, et al. The human vaccines project: a roadmap for cancer vaccine development. Sci Transl Med. 2016;8:334ps9.
26. Nakatsura T, Komori H, Kubo T, Yoshitake Y, Senju S, Katagiri T, et al. Mouse homologue of a novel human Oncofetal antigen, Glypican-3, evokes T-cell–mediated tumor rejection without autoimmune reactions in mice. Clin Cancer Res. 2004;10:8630–40.
27. Komori H, Nakatsura T, Senju S, Yoshitake Y, Motomura Y, Ikuta Y, et al. Identification of HLA-A2- or HLA-A24-restricted CTL epitopes possibly useful for Glypican-3-specific immunotherapy of hepatocellular carcinoma. Clin Cancer Res. 2006;12:2689–97.

28. Sawada Y, Yoshikawa T, Ofuji K, Yoshimura M, Tsuchiya N, Takahashi M, et al. Phase II study of the GPC3-derived peptide vaccine as an adjuvant therapy for hepatocellular carcinoma patients. OncoImmunology. 2016;5:e1129483.
29. Sawada Y, Yoshikawa T, Fujii S, Mitsunaga S, Nobuoka D, Mizuno S, et al. Remarkable tumor lysis in a hepatocellular carcinoma patient immediately following glypican-3-derived peptide vaccination: an autopsy case. Hum Vaccin Immunother. 2013;9:1228–33.
30. Sayem MA, Tomita Y, Yuno A, Hirayama M, Irie A, Tsukamoto H, et al. Identification of glypican-3-derived long peptides activating both CD8+ and CD4+ T cells; prolonged overall survival in cancer patients with Th cell response. OncoImmunology. 2016;5:e1062209.
31. Kagamu H, Shu S. Purification of L-Selectinlow cells promotes the generation of highly potent CD4 antitumor effector T lymphocytes. J Immunol. 1998;160:3444–52.
32. Hu H-M, Winter H, Urba WJ, Fox BA. Divergent roles for CD4+ T cells in the priming and effector/memory phases of adoptive immunotherapy. J Immunol. 2000;165:4246–53.
33. Ma C, Kesarwala AH, Eggert T, Medina-Echeverz J, Kleiner DE, Jin P, et al. NAFLD causes selective CD4+ T lymphocyte loss and promotes hepatocarcinogenesis. Nature. 2016;531:253–7.
34. Toes RE, Blom RJ, Offringa R, Kast WM, Melief CJ. Enhanced tumor outgrowth after peptide vaccination. Functional deletion of tumor-specific CTL induced by peptide vaccination can lead to the inability to reject tumors. J Immunol. 1996;156:3911–8.
35. Toes RE, Offringa R, Blom RJ, Melief CJ, Kast WM. Peptide vaccination can lead to enhanced tumor growth through specific T-cell tolerance induction. Proc Natl Acad Sci. 1996;93:7855–60.
36. Toes REM, van der Voort EIH, Schoenberger SP, Drijfhout JW, van Bloois L, Storm G, et al. Enhancement of tumor outgrowth through CTL Tolerization after peptide vaccination is avoided by peptide presentation on dendritic cells. J Immunol. 1998;160:4449–56.
37. Rahma OE, Ashtar E, Czystowska M, Szajnik ME, Wieckowski E, Bernstein S, et al. A gynecologic oncology group phase II trial of two p53 peptide vaccine approaches: subcutaneous injection and intravenous pulsed dendritic cells in high recurrence risk ovarian cancer patients. Cancer Immunol Immunother. 2012;61:373–84.
38. Srinivasan M, Domanico SZ, Kaumaya PTP, Pierce SK. Peptides of 23 residues or greater are required to stimulate a high affinity class II-restricted T cell response. Eur J Immunol. 1993;23:1011–6.
39. den Boer AT, Diehl L, van GJD M, van der EIH V, Fransen MF, Krimpenfort P, et al. Longevity of antigen presentation and activation status of APC are decisive factors in the balance between CTL immunity versus tolerance. J Immunol. 2001;167:2522–8.
40. Iwama T, Uchida T, Sawada Y, Tsuchiya N, Sugai S, Fujinami N, et al. Vaccination with liposome-coupled glypican-3-derived epitope peptide stimulates cytotoxic T lymphocytes and inhibits GPC3-expressing tumor growth in mice. Biochem Biophys Res Commun. 2016;469:138–43.
41. Phung Y, Gao W, Man Y-G, Nagata S, Ho M. High-affinity monoclonal antibodies to cell surface tumor antigen glypican-3 generated through a combination of peptide immunization and flow cytometry screening. MAbs. 2012;4:592–9.
42. Zhang Y-F, Ho M. Humanization of high-affinity antibodies targeting glypican-3 in hepatocellular carcinoma. Sci Rep. 2016;6:33878.
43. Feng M, Gao W, Wang R, Chen W, Man Y-G, Figg WD, et al. Therapeutically targeting glypican-3 via a conformation-specific single-domain antibody in hepatocellular carcinoma. Proc Natl Acad Sci. 2013;110:E1083–E91.
44. Gao W, Tang Z, Zhang Y-F, Feng M, Qian M, Dimitrov DS, et al. Immunotoxin targeting glypican-3 regresses liver cancer via dual inhibition of Wnt signalling and protein synthesis. Nat Commun. 2015;6:6536.
45. Gao W, Kim H, Feng M, Phung Y, Xavier CP, Rubin JS, et al. Inactivation of Wnt signaling by a human antibody that recognizes the heparan sulfate chains of glypican-3 for liver cancer therapy. Hepatology. 2014;60:576–87.

46. Gao W, Xu Y, Liu J, Ho M. Epitope mapping by a Wnt-blocking antibody: evidence of the Wnt binding domain in heparan sulfate. Sci Rep. 2016;6:26245.
47. Golabi M, Leung A, Lopez C. Simpson-Golabi-Behmel syndrome type 1. In: Pagon RA, Adam MP, Ardinger HH, editors. Gene reviews. Seattle: University of Washington; 2006 Dec 19 [Updated 2011 Jun 23].
48. Sun CK, Chua M-S, He J, So SK. Suppression of glypican 3 inhibits growth of hepatocellular carcinoma cells through up-regulation of TGF-β2. Neoplasia. 2011;13:IN25. (New York, NY)
49. Feng M, Kim H, Phung Y, Ho M. Recombinant soluble glypican 3 protein inhibits the growth of hepatocellular carcinoma in vitro. Int J Cancer. 2011;128:2246–7.
50. Bengochea A, de Souza MM, Lefrancois L, Le Roux E, Galy O, Chemin I, et al. Common dysregulation of Wnt/frizzled receptor elements in human hepatocellular carcinoma. Br J Cancer. 2008;99:143–50.
51. Capurro MI, Xiang Y-Y, Lobe C, Filmus J. Glypican-3 promotes the growth of hepatocellular carcinoma by stimulating canonical Wnt signaling. Cancer Res. 2005;65:6245–54.
52. Capurro M, Martin T, Shi W, Filmus J. Glypican-3 binds to frizzled and plays a direct role in the stimulation of canonical Wnt signaling. J Cell Sci. 2014;127:1565–75.
53. Gao W, Kim H, Ho M. Human monoclonal antibody targeting the Heparan sulfate chains of Glypican-3 inhibits HGF-mediated migration and motility of hepatocellular carcinoma cells. PLoS One. 2015;10:e0137664.
54. Midorikawa Y, Ishikawa S, Iwanari H, Imamura T, Sakamoto H, Miyazono K, et al. Glypican-3, overexpressed in hepatocellular carcinoma, modulates FGF2 and BMP-7 signaling. Int J Cancer. 2003;103:455–65.
55. Cheng W, Tseng C-J, Lin TTC, Cheng I, Pan H-W, Hsu H-C, et al. Glypican-3-mediated oncogenesis involves the insulin-like growth factor-signaling pathway. Carcinogenesis. 2008;29:1319–26.
56. Capurro MI, Xu P, Shi W, Li F, Jia A, Filmus J. Glypican-3 inhibits hedgehog signaling during development by competing with patched for hedgehog binding. Dev Cell. 2008;14:700–11.
57. Cho H-S, Ahn J-M, Han H-J, Cho J-Y. Glypican 3 binds to GLUT1 and decreases glucose transport activity in hepatocellular carcinoma cells. J Cell Biochem. 2010;111:1252–9.
58. Taguchi A, Emoto M, Okuya S, Fukuda N, Nakamori Y, Miyazaki M, et al. Identification of Glypican3 as a novel GLUT4-binding protein. Biochem Biophys Res Commun. 2008;369:1204–8.
59. Capurro MI, Shi W, Filmus J. LRP1 mediates the Shh-induced endocytosis of the GPC3-Shh complex. J Cell Sci. 2012;125:3380–9.
60. Capurro M, Shi W, Izumikawa T, Kitagawa H, Filmus J. Processing by convertases is required for Glypican-3-induced inhibition of hedgehog signaling. J Biol Chem. 2015;290:7576–85.
61. Ishiguro T, Sugimoto M, Kinoshita Y, Miyazaki Y, Nakano K, Tsunoda H, et al. Anti-glypican 3 antibody as a potential antitumor agent for human liver cancer. Cancer Res. 2008;68:9832–8.
62. Kaymakcalan Z, Ibraghimov A, Goodearl AG, Salfeld AJG. Aspects of isotype selection. In: Kontermann R, Dubel S, editors. Antibody engineering. Berlin/Heidelberg: Springer; 2010. p. 291–306.
63. Takai H, Kato A, Kinoshita Y, Ishiguro T, Takai Y, Ohtani Y, et al. Histopathological analyses of the antitumor activity of anti-glypican-3 antibody (GC33) in human liver cancer xenograft models: the essential role of macrophages. Cancer Biol Ther. 2009;8:930–8.
64. Zhu AX, Gold PJ, El-Khoueiry AB, Abrams TA, Morikawa H, Ohishi N, et al. First-in-man phase I study of GC33, a novel recombinant humanized antibody against Glypican-3, in patients with advanced hepatocellular carcinoma. Clin Cancer Res. 2013;19:920–8.
65. Ikeda M, Ohkawa S, Okusaka T, Mitsunaga S, Kobayashi S, Morizane C, et al. Japanese phase I study of GC33, a humanized antibody against glypican-3 for advanced hepatocellular carcinoma. Cancer Sci. 2014;105:455–62.
66. Yen C-J, Daniele B, Kudo M, Merle P, Park J-W, Ross PJ, et al. Randomized phase II trial of intravenous RO5137382/GC33 at 1600 mg every other week and placebo in previously treated patients with unresectable advanced hepatocellular carcinoma (HCC; NCT01507168). 2014. J Clin Oncol. 32 p 4102.

67. Hanaoka H, Nakajima T, Sato K, Watanabe R, Phung Y, Gao W, et al. Photoimmunotherapy of hepatocellular carcinoma-targeting Glypican-3 combined with nanosized albumin-bound paclitaxel. Nanomedicine. 2015;10:1139–47. (London, England)
68. Hanaoka H, Nagaya T, Sato K, Nakamura Y, Watanabe R, Harada T, et al. Glypican-3 targeted human heavy chain antibody as a drug carrier for hepatocellular carcinoma therapy. Mol Pharm. 2015;12:2151–7.
69. FitzGerald DJ, Kreitman R, Wilson W, Squires D, Pastan I. Recombinant immunotoxins for treating cancer. Int J Med Microbiol. 2004;293:577–82.
70. Kreitman RJ, Pastan I. Antibody fusion proteins: anti-CD22 recombinant immunotoxin Moxetumomab Pasudotox. Clin Cancer Res. 2011;17:6398–405.
71. Hassan R, Miller AC, Sharon E, Thomas A, Reynolds JC, Ling A, et al. Major cancer regressions in mesothelioma after treatment with an anti-Mesothelin immunotoxin and immune suppression. Sci Transl Med. 2013;5:208ra147.
72. Mazor R, Onda M, Pastan I. Immunogenicity of therapeutic recombinant immunotoxins. Immunol Rev. 2016;270:152–64.
73. Kreitman RJ. Immunoconjugates and new molecular targets in hairy cell leukemia. ASH Edu Program Book. 2012;2012:660–6.
74. Siegall CB, Haggerty HG, Warner GL, Chace D, Mixan B, Linsley PS, et al. Prevention of immunotoxin-induced immunogenicity by coadministration with CTLA4Ig enhances antitumor efficacy. J Immunol. 1997;159:5168–73.
75. Meister S, Schubert U, Neubert K, Herrmann K, Burger R, Gramatzki M, et al. Extensive immunoglobulin production sensitizes myeloma cells for proteasome inhibition. Cancer Res. 2007;67:1783–92.
76. Onda M, Ghoreschi K, Steward-Tharp S, Thomas C, O'Shea JJ, Pastan IH, et al. Tofacitinib suppresses antibody responses to protein therapeutics in murine hosts. J Immunol. 2014;193:48–55.
77. Manning ML, Mason-Osann E, Onda M, Pastan I. Bortezomib reduces pre-existing antibodies to recombinant immunotoxins in mice. J Immunol. 2015;194:1695–701.
78. Kreitman RJ, Stetler-Stevenson M, Jaffe ES, Conlon KC, Steinberg SM, Wilson W, et al. Complete remissions of adult T-cell leukemia with anti-CD25 recombinant immunotoxin LMB-2 and chemotherapy to block immunogenicity. Clin Cancer Res. 2016;22:310–8.
79. Azemar M, Djahansouzi S, Jäger E, Solbach C, Schmidt M, Maurer AB, et al. Regression of cutaneous tumor lesions in patients Intratumorally injected with a recombinant single-chain antibody-toxin targeted to ErbB2/HER2. Breast Cancer Res Treat. 2003;82:155–64.
80. Weber F, Asher A, Bucholz R, Berger M, Prados M, Chang S, et al. Safety, tolerability, and tumor response of IL4-pseudomonas exotoxin (NBI-3001) in patients with recurrent malignant glioma. J Neuro-Oncol. 2003;64:125–37.
81. Kowalski M, Entwistle J, Cizeau J, Niforos D, Loewen S, Chapman W, et al. A phase I study of an intravesically administered immunotoxin targeting EpCAM for the treatment of nonmuscle-invasive bladder cancer in BCGrefractory and BCG-intolerant patients. Drug Des Devel Ther. 2010;4:313–20.
82. Llovet JM, Real MI, Montaña X, Planas R, Coll S, Aponte J, et al. Arterial embolisation or chemoembolisation versus symptomatic treatment in patients with unresectable hepatocellular carcinoma: a randomised controlled trial. Lancet. 2002;359:1734–9.
83. Roscoe DM, Pai LH, Pastan I. Identification of epitopes on a mutant form of pseudomonas exotoxin using serum from humans treated with pseudomonas exotoxin containing immunotoxins. Eur J Immunol. 1997;27:1459–68.
84. Onda M, Nagata S, FitzGerald DJ, Beers R, Fisher RJ, Vincent JJ, et al. Characterization of the B cell epitopes associated with a truncated form of pseudomonas exotoxin (PE38) used to make immunotoxins for the treatment of cancer patients. J Immunol. 2006;177:8822–34.
85. Onda M, Beers R, Xiang L, Nagata S, Wang Q-c, Pastan I. An immunotoxin with greatly reduced immunogenicity by identification and removal of B cell epitopes. Proc Natl Acad Sci. 2008;105:11311–6.

86. Siegel DL. Translational applications of antibody phage display. Immunol Res. 2008;42:118–31.
87. Liu-Chittenden Y, Huang B, Shim JS, Chen Q, Lee SJ, Anders RA, et al. Genetic and pharmacological disruption of the TEAD-YAP complex suppresses the oncogenic activity of YAP. Genes Dev. 2012;26:1300–5.
88. Mazor R, Vassall AN, Eberle JA, Beers R, Weldon JE, Venzon DJ, et al. Identification and elimination of an immunodominant T-cell epitope in recombinant immunotoxins based on pseudomonas exotoxin a. Proc Natl Acad Sci. 2012;109:E3597–E603.
89. Mazor R, Eberle JA, Hu X, Vassall AN, Onda M, Beers R, et al. Recombinant immunotoxin for cancer treatment with low immunogenicity by identification and silencing of human T-cell epitopes. Proc Natl Acad Sci. 2014;111:8571–6.
90. Mazor R, Crown D, Addissie S, Jang Y, Kaplan G, Pastan I. Elimination of murine and human T-cell epitopes in recombinant immunotoxin eliminates neutralizing and anti-drug antibodies in vivo. Cell Mol Immunol. 2015;14(5):432–42.
91. Mazor R, Zhang J, Xiang L, Addissie S, Awuah P, Beers R, et al. Recombinant immunotoxin with T-cell epitope mutations that greatly reduce immunogenicity for treatment of Mesothelin-expressing tumors. Mol Cancer Ther. 2015;14:2789–96.
92. Wang C, Gao W, Feng M, Pastan I, Ho M. Construction of an immunotoxin, HN3-mPE24, targeting glypican-3 for liver cancer therapy. Oncotarget. 2016;5
93. Hashimoto K, Perera A, Ogita Y, Nakamura M, Ishiguro T, Sano Y, et al. A phase I dose escalation and cohort expansion study of T-cell redirecting bispecific antibody against Glypican 3 in patients with advanced solid tumors. 2016 ASCO annual meeting. J Clin Oncol. 2016; 34. p suppl; abstr TPS2592.
94. Jackson HJ, Rafiq S, Brentjens RJ. Driving CAR T-cells forward. Nat Rev Clin Oncol. 2016;13:370–83.
95. Kalos M, Levine BL, Porter DL, Katz S, Grupp SA, Bagg A, et al. T cells with chimeric antigen receptors have potent antitumor effects and can establish memory in patients with advanced leukemia. Sci Transl Med. 2011;3(95):95ra73.
96. van der Stegen SJC, Hamieh M, Sadelain M. The pharmacology of second-generation chimeric antigen receptors. Nat Rev Drug Discov. 2015;14:499–509.
97. Carpenito C, Milone MC, Hassan R, Simonet JC, Lakhal M, Suhoski MM, et al. Control of large, established tumor xenografts with genetically retargeted human T cells containing CD28 and CD137 domains. Proc Natl Acad Sci. 2009;106:3360–5.
98. Zhong X-S, Matsushita M, Plotkin J, Riviere I, Sadelain M. Chimeric antigen receptors combining 4-1BB and CD28 signaling domains augment PI3kinase/AKT/Bcl-XL activation and CD8+ T cell-mediated tumor eradication. Mol Ther. 2009;18:413–20.
99. Gao H, Li K, Tu H, Pan X, Jiang H, Shi B, et al. Development of T cells redirected to Glypican-3 for the treatment of hepatocellular carcinoma. Clin Cancer Res. 2014;20:6418–28.
100. Giakoustidis A, Giakoustidis D, Mudan S, Sklavos A, Williams R. Molecular signalling in hepatocellular carcinoma: role of and crosstalk among WNT/ss-catenin, sonic hedgehog, notch and Dickkopf-1. Can J Gastroenterol Hepatol. 2015;29:209–17.
101. Li W, Guo L, Rathi P, Marinova E, Gao X, Wu M-F, et al. Redirecting T cells to Glypican-3 with 4-1BB.ζ CAR results in Th-1 polarization and potent anti-tumor activity. Hum Gene Ther. 2016;28(5):437–48.
102. Li W, Guo L, Rathi P, Marinova E, Gao X, Wu MF, et al. Redirecting T cells to Glypican-3 with 4-1BB zeta chimeric antigen receptors results in Th1 polarization and potent antitumor activity. Hum Gene Ther. 2016;28(5):437–48.
103. Trinh TL, Wu Q, Chang L-J, Ho M, Liu C. GPC3-specific chimeric antigen receptor T cell in combination with Sorafenib as a novel therapeutic treatment for hepatocellular carcinoma. New Orleans/Philadelphia: AACR; 2016, April 16–20. Cancer Res. p Abstract nr 2316.
104. Dargel C, Bassani-Sternberg M, Hasreiter J, Zani F, Bockmann J-H, Thiele F, et al. T cells engineered to express a T-cell receptor specific for Glypican-3 to recognize and kill hepatoma cells in vitro and in mice. Gastroenterology. 2015;149:1042–52.

Chapter 8
Immune Suppressor Mechanisms in HCC

Tim F. Greten and Firouzeh Korangy

8.1 The Liver –a Tolerogenic Organ?

The liver has been recognized as a tolerogenic organ for many years. Early liver transplantation studies in outbred pigs conduced in the 1960s demonstrated a long-term allograft survival without immunosuppression in 12/55 pigs [1]. Long-term follow-up of liver transplanted patients revealed a similar phenomenon. The Starzl group reported that they were able to wean 29% of their patients from immunosuppression for an average of 10.8 year [2]. In addition, it should be noted that the specific anatomy of the liver with two feeding vessel represents another challenge for the liver. Only 20% of the blood supply to the liver stems from the hepatic artery, while approximately 80% of the blood supply to the liver comes from the portal vein, which drains the entire gastrointestinal tract and is loaded with so called microbial associated molecular patterns (MAMPS) such as LPS, which are capable of inducing massive immune responses [3, 4].

Thus, the liver has to be equipped with special mechanisms leading to liver-induced tolerance. It is beyond the scope of this chapter to cover all studies and potential mechanism leading to liver induced tolerance, which have been covered by a number of excellent reviews in the past [5–7]. However, there are a few important points, which need to be made to better understand immune suppressor mechanism in HCC.

The liver provides a unique immunological environment. Liver sinusoidal endothelial cells (LSEC) cover hepatic vessels. LSEC represent fenestrated cellular barriers between sinusoidal blood and hepatocytes. They sample blood, which contains nutrients and microbial antigen from the gut and induce T cell tolerance to antigens to which no preexisting immunity exists [8]. LSECs express toll like receptors (TLR), MHC class I and II molecules. They can function as antigen presenting cells

T.F. Greten (✉) • F. Korangy
GI Malignancy Section, TGIB, Center for Cancer Research, NCI, Bethesda, MD, USA
e-mail: gretentf@mail.nih.gov

T.F. Greten (ed.), *Immunotherapy of Hepatocellular Carcinoma*,
DOI 10.1007/978-3-319-64958-0_8

together with liver resident macrophages (Kupffer cells), hepatic stellate cells, and dendritic cells. Innate immune cells such as NK, NKT and γ/δ T cells can be found at much higher frequency in the liver than in peripheral blood. Expression of immunosuppressive cytokines (IL-4, IL-10 and TGF-β) has been reported along with an accumulation of Foxp3$^+$ regulatory T cells and expression of B7-H1 in transplantation setting [5]. Hepatomas variably express MHC class I molecules but no MHC class II and have low levels of the costimulatory molecules CD80 and CD86 on their surface [9, 10].

8.1.1 Chronic Inflammation Leading to Immunosuppression and T Cell Exhaustion

Chronic liver inflammation induced by non-alcoholic steatohepatitis (NASH) or viral hepatitis can progress to liver cirrhosis and eventually to carcinomas [11]. Genetic and epigenetic changes observed in HCC may be the results of chronic inflammation leading to the expression of novel tumor antigens and/or deregulation of the expression of oncofetal and cancer testis antigen including alpha-fetoprotein, glypican-3, NY-ESO.1, members of the MAGE gene family and others [12] (see also chapter xxx). NY-ESO is a cancer testis antigen, which is expressed in 25% of all HCC cases [13]. We studied serum and PBMC samples from HCC patients. We found NY-ESO-specific antibodies in 23/189 screened HCC patients, which correlated with course of the disease (Fig. 8.1).

Flowcytometry analysis revealed NY-ESO-specific CD4$^+$ and CD8$^+$ T cell responses in HCC patients, who did not receive any type of an immune-related therapy clearly indicating that tumor-specific humoral and cellular immune response can be found in patients with HCC. Similar studies have been published from colleagues in the field: The Thimme group used overlapping peptides spanning the entire alpha-fetoprotein (AFP), glypican-3 (GPC-3), melanoma-associated gene-A1 (MAGE-A1) and New York-esophageal squamous cell carcinoma-1 (NY-ESO-1) proteins and MAGE-1 and AFP-tetramers to study naturally occurring CD8$^+$ T cell responses in a large cohort of HCC patients in the periphery and as well as in tumor tissues. Naturally occurring tumor-specific T cell responses were present in patients with HCC and correlated with patient survival [12] (Fig. 8.2).

Similar results were published by Wada and colleagues and from He's group. As early as 1998 Wada et al. described that an infiltration of resected tumors by CD3$^+$ T lymphocytes correlated with improved survival [14]. A recent study from He's group corroborated this data and found that PD-L1 staining correlated with CD3$^+$ and CD8$^+$ T cell densities in tumors and could be used to predict recurrence rates [15]. Interestingly, a number of different treatments currently being used as standard of care either induce or enhance tumor-specific immune responses in patients with HCC. Mizokushi et al. evaluated T cell responses in HCC patients undergoing RFA. These investigators observed immune responses to antigens for which no T cell

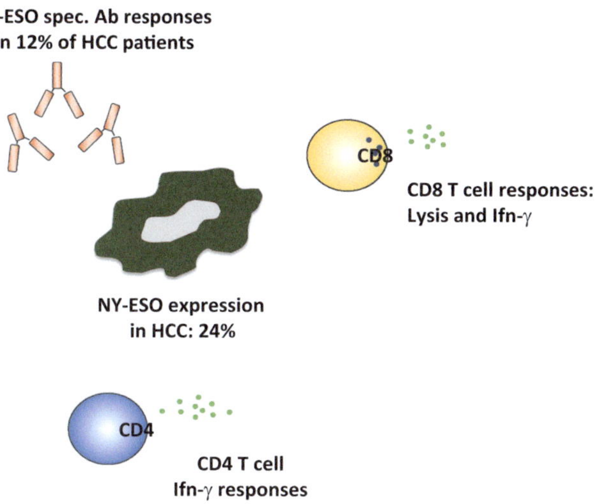

Fig. 8.1 Humoral and cellular NY-ESO specific immune responses can be found in patients with HCC [13]

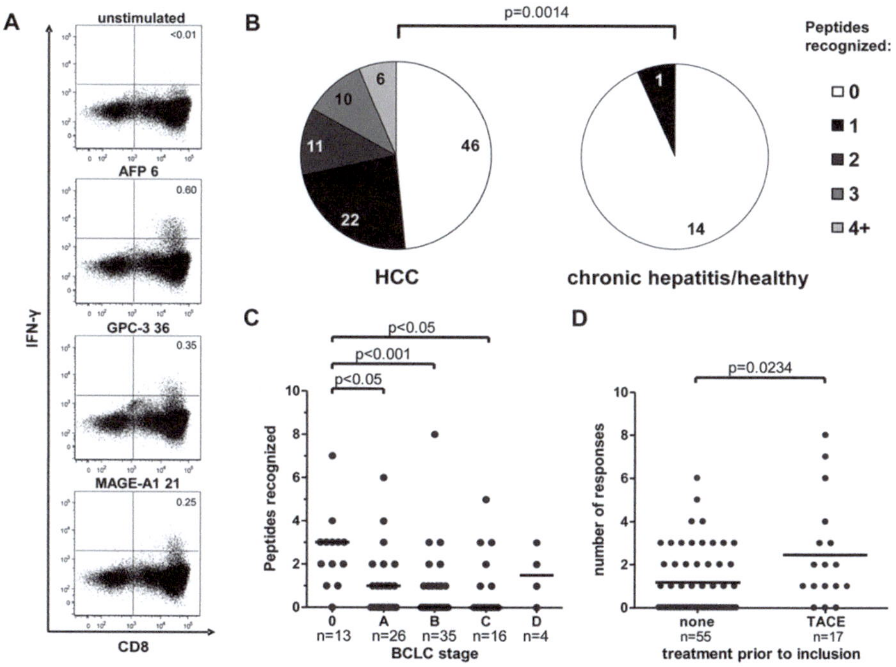

Fig. 8.2 Tumor-specific T cell responses are found in patients with HCC [12]

response was detected at baseline prior to RFA and the number of tumor-specific T cells after RFA correlated with the prevention of HCC recurrence in patients treated with curative intent [16]. Ayaru et al. evaluated immune responses in 10 HCC patients undergoing TACE. He noticed an expansion of AFP-specific CD4 T cell responses upon TACE treatment. Interestingly, patients with increased frequencies of AFP-specific CD4 T cells after treatment also demonstrated more tumor necrosis and an improved clinical outcome [17]. While the majority of studies have focused on CD8+ T cell responses only few investigators studied CD4 T cell responses. Fu and colleagues studied the role of cytotoxic CD4 T cells in 547 HCC patients [18]. Both circulating and liver-infiltrating $CD4^+$ CTLs were found to be significantly increased in HCC patients during early stage disease, but decreased in progressive stages of HCC. $CD4^+$ CTL loss correlated with worse clinical outcome. A more in depth analysis of tumor-specific immune responses to ablative therapies can be found in [19].

How can tumors progress in presence of tumor specific immune responses? One possible explanation comes from the Thimme group, who showed that Interferon-γ production by antigen-specific T cells in patients with HCC was impaired. As a matter of fact the presence of antigen specific T cells in patients with different types of cancer has been observed for many years and one of possible explanation how tumors evade tumor specific immune responses is basd on some very elegant work from Robert Schreiber, who described the *"Cancer immunoediting concept"*.

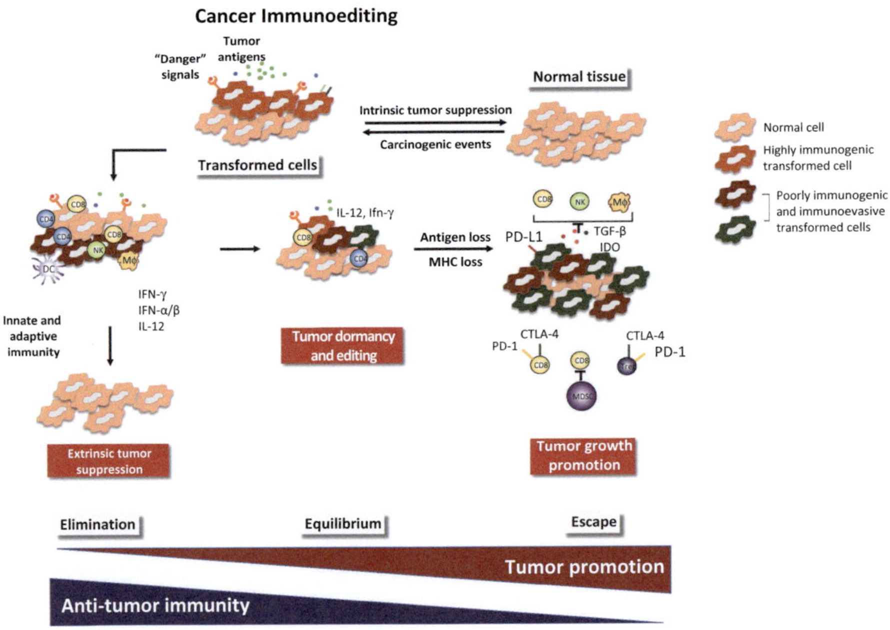

The cancer immunoediting concept modified from [20]

Cancer immunoediting consists of three sequential phases: elimination, equilibrium, and escape. Early immunological mechanisms (innate and adaptive responses) lead to the elimination of cancer, however a few cancer cells may survive this process and may go into the equilibrium phase, in which immune responses (mainly adaptive responses) prevent outgrowth of existing tumors. However, constant immune selection pressure placed on genetically unstable tumor cells held in equilibrium may fuel the outgrowth of tumor cell variants that (i) are either no longer recognized by adaptive immunity (ii) become insensitive to immune effector mechanisms, or (iii) induce an immunosuppressive state within the tumor microenvironment. Tumors, which have entered the escape phase are no longer controlled by innate or adaptive immune responses and become clinically apparent. In this chapter we will describe different mechanisms that HCC have specifically developed to escape adaptive and innate immune responses.

8.2 Cell Mediated Immune Suppressor Mechanisms

8.2.1 Myeloid Derived Suppressor Cells (MDSC)

MDSC are one of the major components of the tumor microenvironment. The characteristic feature of these cells is their potent immune suppressive activity [21]. As a matter of fact, MDSC are defined by their suppressive activity [22]. A number of different mechanisms have been described how MDSC can suppress effector function: The two best described mechanism rely on either arginase expression, which will deprive T cells of the amino acid arginine. Arginine is necessary for T cell proliferation or production of ROS, which can impair adaptive immune responses. MDSC have the ability to support tumor progression by promoting tumor cell survival, angiogenesis, invasion of healthy tissue by tumor cells, and metastases [23]. MDSC are generated in the bone marrow and, in tumor- bearing hosts, migrate to peripheral lymphoid organs and the tumor to contribute to the formation of the tumor microenvironment [24]. Accumulation of MDSC is mediated by tumor-secreted cytokines and/or chemokines [22]. G-CSF, GM-CSF, IL-6, CCL2 and VEGF are commonly found in tumor bearing hosts and also cause MDSC expansion in HCC bearing mice [25, 26] and humans [27].

There are two different types of MDSC, as identified in studies in both mice and humans: polymorphonuclear MDSC (PMN-MDSC) are morphologically and phenotypically similar to neutrophils, whereas monocytic MDSC (M-MDSC) are similar to monocytes [28, 29]. In 2008 we described a population of CD14^{+}HLA-DR^{lo} cells, which accumulated in peripheral blood and tumors of patients with HCC. These cells suppressed proliferation and cytokine production of T cells and induced Foxp3^{+} regulatory T cells *in vitro* [30]. In further studies we were able to demonstrate that human MDSC also suppress NK cell function *in vitro* [31]. Interestingly, we were able to recapitulate this observation recently in a murine HCC model when studying cellular senescence [25]. Cellular senescence is the phenomenon by which normal diploid cells cease to divide. Different inducers of cellular senescence are known including DNA damage in response to elevated reactive oxygen species (ROS), activation of oncogenes and cell-cell fusion. An increase of cellular senescence has been described in the liver of patients with different types of liver diseases [32]. We studied the effect of oncogene induced senescence in the liver of mice and found that senescent cells cause CCR2/CCL2 dependent an accumulation of imature myeloid cells, which in the presence of tumors remained imature and suppressed NK cell function accelerating HCC growth. Results confirming this observation were made, when we studied senescence markers, myeloid cells and NK cells in peri-tumoral tissue samples from HCC patients. Here, we could demonstrate that patients, who displayed a genetic signature resulting in cellular senescence in the tumor microenvironment also had more myeloid cells, less activation of NK cells and an impaired outcome [25]. An accumulation of MDSC in HCC patients has been reported by different experts in the field in different clinical settings. $CD14^{+}HLA\text{-}DR^{lo}$ cells correlated with early recurrence after resection [33], hepatic arterial infusion chemotherapy [34], radiation [35] and tumor progression [27].

Approaches to deplete MDSC include low-dose gemcitabine and 5-fluorouracil treatment and approaches to inhibit their immunosuppressive function include molecules that interfere with ROS and NO production by MDSC, such as PDE-5 inhibitors and nitric-oxide-releasing aspririn [36]. More recently, approaches targeting Gr-1, CSF-1R, CCR2, CXCR2 and STAT3 are being evaluated (some of them in clinical trials in non-HCC malignancies).

Activated hepatic stellate cells (HSC) have been reported to induce and immunosuppressive environment and are associated with poor clinical outcome [37]. Upon activation HSC skew monocytes from an inflammatory to an immunosuppressive phenotype and induce features of aggressive growth of HCC in cells. This HSC monocyte interaction results in early tumor recurrence and poor survival of liver cancer patients. Moreover they can induce the contact dependent accumulation of MDSC either through CD44 on HSC or through hydrogen peroxide depletion by catalase [38, 39]. HSC can also directly trigger T cell dysfunction through pathways analogues to other immunosuppressive cells. They are capable of inducing T cell apoptosis through PD-L1 expression [40].

8.2.2 Regulatory T Cells (Tregs)

Regulatory T cells (Tregs) are mainly known for their pivotal role in the context if autoimmune diseases. Absence of Tregs leads to massive autoimmune diseases [41]. Tregs have been found to accumulate in the environment of multiple different tumors [42]. Tregs can be identified by flowcytometry. They are $CD4^{+}CD25^{hi}$, $CD127^{lo}$, $Foxp3^{+}$, $CTLA4^{+}$ and $CCR4^{+}$. They inhibit immune responses through various mechanisms: CD25 depletes IL-2, CTLA-4 competeswith CD28 on T cells and downregulation of CD80 and CD86 through CTLA-4. Tregs can express TGF-β and IL-10 and produce adenosine through CD39 and CD37, which they express on their surface. Tumor cell secreted IL-1α induces CCL22 and the recruitment of regulatory T cells in HCC [43].

We first described an accumulation of Tregs in patients with HCC in 2005 [44]. Similar results have been described by others [45]. A correlation of tumor infiltrating Tregs and intra-tumoral macrophages has been described in HCC [46]. Two studies found a correlation between the presence of intra-tumoral Tregs and clinical outcome. Fu and colleagues described a significant increase in the frequency of circulating $CD4^{+}CD25^{+}FoxP3^{+}$ Treg in patients with HCC. They observed an abundant accumulation of Tregs concurrent with significantly reduced infiltration of $CD8^{+}$ T cells in tumors but not in non-tumor regions. Expression of granzyme A, granzyme B, and perforin was decreased dramatically in tumor-infiltrating $CD8^{+}$ T cells and an increased quantity of circulating Treg was associated with high mortality and reduced survival time of HCC patients [47]. Around the same time Gao and and colleagues described that the balance between $CD8^{+}$ cytotoxic T cells and intratumoral $CD4^{+}$ Tregs was an independent prognostic factor for overall survival [48].

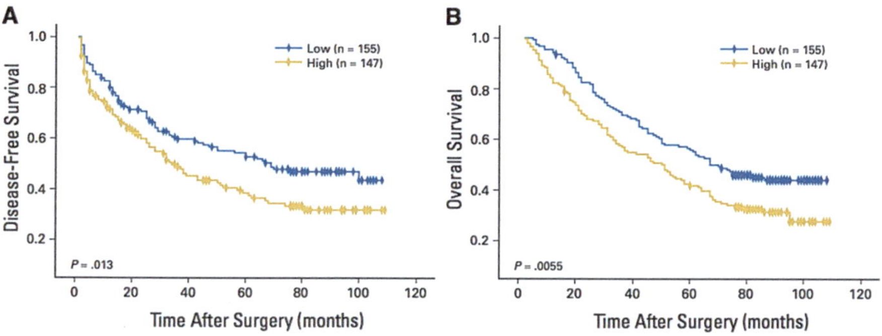

Kaplan-Meier analysis of disease-free survival and overall survival for (**a** and **b**) depending on the presence of tumor-infiltrating regulatory T cells (Tregs) [48]

More recently Kalathil et al. demonstrated an accumulation of Tregs, exhausted T helper ($PD1^{+}$ CD4 T cells) cells, MDSC as well as an impaired IFN-γ production and granzyme release by T cells from HCC patients [49]. Assuming that an elimination of regulatory T cells in patients with HCC may enhance tumor-specific immune responses we studied the effect of Treg depletion *in vitro*. As expected, we could unmaks AFP-specific T cell responses in vitro after depletion of Tregs from PBMC of HCC patients [50]. Based on this data we performed a small proof of concept study in patients with advanced HCC ineligible for any other type of HCC specific therapy and treated these patients with low dose cyclophosphamide in an attempt to specifically target Tregs. It had been shown that low dose cyclophoshamide treatment eliminates Tregs [51] and we tested whether Treg depletion would enhance anti-tumor immunity in HCC patients. As predicted based on our preclinical data, we were able to demonstrate enhanced immune responses in HCC patients treated with low dose cyclophosphamide [50]. The possible impact on Tregs by sorafenib was reported in small cohort of 19 HCC, but this data still needs to be confirmed by others [52]. The role of $CD8^+FoxP3^+$ regulatory T cells in HCC has been studied by Yang et al. [53]. The frequency of $CD8^+FoxP3^+$ regulatory T cells was higher in HCC patients compared to healthy control donors. $CD8^+FoxP3^+$ regulatory T cells displayed an activated phenotype and acted as effector memory cells ($CD45RA^-CCR7^-CD27^{+/-}CD28^+$). Finally, a higher percentage of intrahepatic $CD8^+FoxP3^+$ regulatory T cells was found in patients with advanced HCC than in those with early HCC.

8.2.3 Macrophages

Hepatic macrophages consist of liver resident Kupffer cells, which are originated from the fetal yolk-sack, and infiltrated bone marrow-derived monocytes/macrophages [54]. The liver harbors about 80% of all macrophages of the body and is furthermore patrolled by blood monocytes [55]. Kupffer cells belong to the reticuloendothelial system in the liver, a highly dynamic and complex network, which constitutes a primary line of defense against invading microorganisms, functions as a sensor for altered tissue integrity and largely contributes to the upkeep of tissue homeostasis [54]. Kupffer cells play a major role in maintaining immunological tolerance in the liver and in providing an anti-inflammatory micromilieu during homeostasis. As such they express high levels of PDL-1, but low levels of costimulatory molecules [56]. PD-L1 expression on Kupffer cells was shown to be increased in tumor tissues compared with surrounding non-tumor liver tissues in patients with HCC and this correlated with poorer survival [57]. $PD\text{-}L1^+$ Kupffer cells co-localize in the tumor stroma with $PD\text{-}1^+$ T cells, which results in decreased proliferative ability and effector function. PD-L1/PD-1 blockade recovered effector T cell function *in vitro* [57]. In a different study Zhu and colleagues investigated whether macrophage-colony stimulating factor (M-CSF) may affect outcome of HCC patients. The group tested M-CSF expression and density of macrophages by immunohistochemistry in tissue microarrays containing paired tumor and peri-tumoral liver tissue from 105 patients who had undergone hepatectomy for histologically proven HCC. Interestingly, neither intra-tumoral M-CSF nor macrophage density was associated with clinical outcome. In contrast high peri-tumoral M-CSF and macrophage density, which correlated with large tumor size, presence of intrahepatic metastasis, and high TNM stage, were independent prognostic factors for both overall survival and disease free survival [58]. M-CSF seems to play an important role in this context. M-CSF can induce an M2 type macrophage. While the differentiation of macrophages into M1 and M2 type macrophages is not as clear as it used to be, M2 macrophages are known decrease inflammation, encourage tissue repair and promote tumor growth. In 2006 Xin Wang's group from the NCI studied the liver environment of patients with HCC and identified a unique inflammation/

immune response related signature consisting of a set of 17 genes, which was associated with increased liver metastasis. This signature contained Th1-like or Th2-like cytokines and CSF-1. Livers bearing metastatic HCC also showed higher CSF-1 gene expression, compared to livers bearing non-metastatic HCC [59].

8.2.4 Other Immune Cells with Suppressor Function

In a recent publication Xiao et al. described a pro-tumorigenic subset of B cells that constitutively expressed higher levels of programmed cell death-1 (PD-1) and constituted about 10% of all B cells in advanced-stage HCC [60]. These cells were able to suppress tumor-specific T-cell immunity upon encountering PD-L1^{+} cells or undergoing PD-1 triggering and promoted cancer growth via IL10 signals. CD14^{+} dendritic cells with immune regulatory function are a different immune cell subset with suppressor function and have been described in patients with HCC by Han et al. [61]. They represent 13% of peripheral blood mononuclear cells and suppress T-cell response through interleukin (IL)-10 and indoleamine-2,3-dioxygenase (IDO). Unexpectedly, CD14^{+} DCs expressed high levels of cytotoxic T-lymphocyte antigen-4 (CTLA-4) and programmed death-1 and therefore may be a target in patients treated with immune checkpoint inhibitors.

Th17 cells are a CD4 T helper subset defined by their production of interleukin 17. These cells play an important role in maintaining mucosal barriers and contributing to pathogen clearance at mucosal surfaces. Their role in the context of cancer remains controversial [62]. We analyzed the phenotype of *in vitro* primed Th17 cells and found that CCR4^{+}CCR6^{+}Th17 cells suppressed the lytic function, proliferation, and cytokine secretion of both Ag-specific and CD3/CD28/CD2-stimulated autologous CD8^{+} T cells. In contrast, CCR4^{-}CCR6^{+} CD4^{+} T cells, which also secrete IL-17, did not affect the CD8^{+} T cells. Analysis of CD4^{+} T cells in peripheral blood from patients with HCC revealed an increase in the frequency of CCR4^{+}CCR6^{+}, but not CCR4^{-}CCR6^{+} Th17 cells in peripheral blood of HCC patients suggesting that these cells may contribute to impairment of CD8^{+} T cell effector functions [63].

Th9 cells represent another CD4 T helper subset. These cells have been described in mice and men and have potent antitumor activity, particular in melanoma [64]. The frequency of IL-9 producing Th9 cells has been reported to be higher in HCC patients compared to healthy controls. Analysis of tumor tissue demonstrated higher frequencies of Th9 cells in tumor and peri-tumor tissues than in unaffected liver. Surprisingly worse outcome correlated with increased Th9 cell frequencies [65].

Cancers rely on the tumor microenvironment, which comprises a variety of non-malignant stromal cells for growth, invasion, and metastasis [66]. Neutrophils can either promote or inhibit tumor progression, depending on the tumor microenvironment, via release of cytokines. Recent evidence has indicated that there is a complex and multidirectional interplay between tumor cells and immune or non-immune stromal cells during cancer development and progression. The interaction between tumor and stromal cells may polarize stromal cells to favor tumor promotion [67].

Multiple studies have been reported on neutrophils and different types of cancer. Using tissue samples, peripheral blood and performing in vitro studies, Han and colleagues demonstrated that tumor associated neutrophils recruit macrophages and Treg cells to HCCs and thereby promote their growth, progression as well as resistance to sorafenib [68].

Tumor-associated fibroblasts (TAFs), which are a major component of the tumor stroma, significantly modify cancer evolution [69] support primary tumor growth through the secretion of various cytokines and growth factors. In the context of HCC, TAF have been shown to release IL-6 and SDF-1a, which induce MDSC generation and activation, and impair anti-tumor immunity. This creates favorable conditions for HCC progression [70].

TIE2-expressing monocytes (TEMs) are a recently described subpopulation of peripheral and tumor-infiltrating myeloid cells presumed to be equipped with profound pro-angiogenic activity; these cells are found both in mice and humans [71–73]. In a study of 168 HCV-infected patients including 89 HCC patients a significant positive correlation was observed between micro-vessel density and frequency of $CD14^{+}CD16^{+}TIE2^{+}$TEMs in the blood or tumors. Frequency of TIE-2 expressing monocytes changed with therapeutic response or recurrence [74].

Cabrera and colleagues demonstrated elevated levels of soluble CD25 levels in HCC patients. Increased serum levels correlated with tumor burden and worse clinical outcome. *In vitro* studies demonstrated that soluble CD25 suppressed effector T cell function [75–77].

8.2.5 Immunosuppressive Molecules

With the recent approval of different immune checkpoint inhibitors such as anti-CTLA4, anti-PD1 and anti-PDL1 these molecules have gained significant interest. A number of retrospective studies using HCC samples have been conducted. PD-L1 expression ranges from 45 to 100% [78–80]. In a cohort of 240 patients with surgically resected HCC, tumoral PD-L1 expression was associated with aggressive clinicopathologic features and a statistically significantly shorter disease-free survival [81]. In contrast a recent study of 65 stage I to IV HCC tissue samples, Gabrielson and colleagues found a correlation between PD-L1 staining and high CD3 and CD8 staining intensity. Here PD-L1 staining predicted lower recurrence rates and prolonged progression free survival [15]. Similar results were described in a retrospective study from Germany [82].

8.2.6 AFP

α-fetoprotein is an oncofetal protein that is highly expressed in abnormalities of prenatal development and several epithelial cancers, including HCC. In HCC patients exhibiting high levels of serum AFP, a lower ratio of myeloid/plasmacytoid circulating DCs compared with patients with low serum AFP levels and healthy donors has been observed. Thus AFP or a cofactor bound to tumor derived AFP may cause dendritic cell dysfunction [83].

8.2.7 NKT Cells

Natural killer T (NKT) cells are a heterogeneous group of T lymphocytes that share properties of both T cells and natural killer cells. NKT cells recognize glycolipid antigens via an invariant TCR -chain and play a central role in various immune responses. Frequencies of V-alpha 24/V-beta 11 iNKT cells are increased in tumors, derived from patients with HCC. In depth studies of tumor derived iNKT cells from HCC patients revealed that the tumor microenvironment of HCC modified the NKT cell repertoire and shifted them towards a subset able to generate Th2 cytokines that can inhibit the expansion of tumor Ag-specific $CD8^+$ T cells. Because CD4 iNKT cells appear inefficient in tumor defense and may even favor tumor growth and recurrence, novel iNKT-targeted therapies should restore CD4 iNKT cells at the tumor site [84].

References

1. Calne RY, Sells RA, Pena JR, Davis DR, Millard PR, Herbertson BM, et al. Induction of immunological tolerance by porcine liver allografts. Nature. 1969;223:472–6.
2. Mazariegos GV, Reyes J, Marino IR, Demetris AJ, Flynn B, Irish W, et al. Weaning of immunosuppression in liver transplant recipients. Transplant. 1997;63:243–9. NIH Public Access
3. Nemeth E, Baird AW, O'Farrelly C. Microanatomy of the liver immune system. Semin Immunopathol. 2009;31:333–43.
4. Caesar R, Reigstad CS, Bäckhed HK, Reinhardt C, Ketonen M, Lundén GÖ, et al. Gut-derived lipopolysaccharide augments adipose macrophage accumulation but is not essential for impaired glucose or insulin tolerance in mice. Gut BMJ Publishing Group. 2012;61:1701–7.
5. Moris D, Lu L, Qian S. Mechanisms of liver-induced tolerance. Curr Opin Organ Transplant. 2016;22(1):71–8.
6. Crispe IN. Immune tolerance in liver disease. Hepatology. 2014;60:2109–17.
7. Heymann F, Tacke F. Immunology in the liver – from homeostasis to disease. Nat Rev Gastroenterol Hepatol. 2016;13:88–110. Nature Publishing Group
8. Thomson AW, Knolle PA. Antigen-presenting cell function in the tolerogenic liver environment. Nat Rev Immunol. 2010;10:753–66. Nature Publishing Group

9. Tatsumi T, Takehara T, Katayama K, Mochizuki K, Yamamoto M, Kanto T, et al. Expression of costimulatory molecules B7–1 (CD80) and B7–2 (CD86) on human hepatocellular carcinoma. Hepatology. 1997;25:1108–14. Wiley Subscription Services, Inc., A Wiley Company
10. Fujiwara K, Higashi T, Nouso K, Nakatsukasa H, Kobayashi Y, Uemura M, et al. Decreased expression of B7 costimulatory molecules and major histocompatibility complex class-I in human hepatocellular carcinoma. J Gastroenterol Hepatol. 2004;19:1121–7. 2004 ed.
11. Forner A, Llovet JM, Bruix J. Hepatocellular carcinoma. Lancet. 2012;379:1245–55.
12. Flecken T, Schmidt N, Hild S, Gostick E, Drognitz O, Zeiser R, et al. Immunodominance and functional alterations of tumor-associated antigen-specific CD8(+) T-cell responses in hepatocellular carcinoma. Hepatology. 2014;59:1415–26.
13. Korangy F, Ormandy LA, Bleck JS, Klempnauer J, Wilkens L, Manns MP, et al. Spontaneous tumor-specific humoral and cellular immune responses to NY-ESO-1 in hepatocellular carcinoma. Clin Cancer Res. 2004;10:4332–41.
14. Wada Y, Nakashima O, Kutami R, Yamamoto O, Kojiro M. Clinicopathological study on hepatocellular carcinoma with lymphocytic infiltration. Hepatology. 1998;27:407–14. WB Saunders
15. Gabrielson A, Wu Y, Wang H, Jiang J, Kallakury B, Gatalica Z, et al. Intratumoral CD3 and CD8 T-cell densities associated with relapse-free survival in HCC. Cancer Immunol Res. 2016;4:419–30. American Association for Cancer Research
16. Mizukoshi E, Yamashita T, Arai K, Sunagozaka H, Ueda T, Arihara F, et al. Enhancement of tumor-associated antigen-specific T cell responses by radiofrequency ablation of hepatocellular carcinoma. Hepatology. 2013;57:1448–57.
17. Ayaru L, Pereira SP, Alisa A, Pathan AA, Williams R, Davidson B, et al. Unmasking of alpha-fetoprotein-specific CD4(+) T cell responses in hepatocellular carcinoma patients undergoing embolization. J Immunol. 2007;178:1914–22.
18. Fu J, Zhang Z, Zhou L, Qi Z, Xing S, Lv J, et al. Impairment of CD4+ cytotoxic T cells predicts poor survival and high recurrence rates in patients with hepatocellular carcinoma. Hepatology. 2013;58:139–49.
19. Greten TF, Duffy AG, Korangy F. Hepatocellular carcinoma from an immunologic perspective. Clin Cancer Res. 2013;19:6678–85.
20. Schreiber RD, Old LJ, Smyth MJ. Cancer Immunoediting: integrating Immunity's roles in cancer suppression and promotion. Science. 2011;331:1565–70.
21. Kumar V, Patel S, Tcyganov E, Gabrilovich DI. The nature of myeloid-derived suppressor cells in the tumor microenvironment. Trends Immunol. 2016;37:208–20.
22. Gabrilovich DI, Nagaraj S. Myeloid-derived suppressor cells as regulators of the immune system. Nat Rev Immunol. 2009;9:162–74.
23. Condamine T, Ramachandran I, Youn J-I, Gabrilovich DI. Regulation of tumor metastasis by myeloid-derived suppressor cells. Annu Rev Med. 2015;66:97–110.
24. Gabrilovich DI, Ostrand-Rosenberg S, Bronte V. Coordinated regulation of myeloid cells by tumours. Nat Rev Immunol. 2012;12:253–68. Nature Publishing Group
25. Eggert T, Wolter K, Ji J, Ma C, Yevsa T, Klotz S, et al. Distinct functions of senescence-associated immune responses in liver tumor surveillance and tumor progression. Cancer Cell. 2016;30:533–47.
26. Kapanadze T, Gamrekelashvili J, Ma C, Chan C, Zhao F, Hewitt S, et al. Regulation of accumulation and function of myeloid derived suppressor cells in different murine models of hepatocellular carcinoma. J Hepatol. 2013;59:1007–13.
27. Arihara F, Mizukoshi E, Kitahara M, Takata Y, Arai K, Yamashita T, et al. Increase in CD14(+) HLA-DR (−/low) myeloid-derived suppressor cells in hepatocellular carcinoma patients and its impact on prognosis. Cancer Immunol Immunother. 2013;62:1421–30.
28. Bronte V, Brandau S, Chen S-H, Colombo MP, Frey AB, Greten TF, et al. Recommendations for myeloid-derived suppressor cell nomenclature and characterization standards. Nat Comms. 2016;7:12150.

29. Greten TF, Manns MP, Korangy F. Myeloid derived suppressor cells in human diseases. Int Immunopharmacol. 2011;11:802–7.
30. Hoechst B, Ormandy LA, Ballmaier M, Lehner F, Krüger C, Manns MP, et al. A new population of myeloid-derived suppressor cells in hepatocellular carcinoma patients induces CD4(+) CD25(+)Foxp3(+) T cells. Gastroenterology. 2008;135:234–43.
31. Hoechst B, Voigtlaender T, Ormandy L, Gamrekelashvili J, Zhao F, Wedemeyer H, et al. Myeloid derived suppressor cells inhibit natural killer cells in patients with hepatocellular carcinoma via the NKp30 receptor. Hepatology. 2009;50:799–807.
32. Wiemann SU, Satyanarayana A, Tsahuridu M, Tillmann HL, Zender L, Klempnauer J, et al. Hepatocyte telomere shortening and senescence are general markers of human liver cirrhosis. FASEB J. 2002;16:935–42.
33. Gao X-H, Tian L, Wu J, Ma X-L, Zhang C-Y, Zhou Y, et al. Circulating CD14 +HLA-DR –/low myeloid-derived suppressor cells predicted early recurrence of hepatocellular carcinoma after surgery. Hepatol Res. 2017;47(10):1061–71.
34. Mizukoshi E, Yamashita T, Arai K, Terashima T, Kitahara M, Nakagawa H, et al. Myeloid-derived suppressor cells correlate with patient outcomes in hepatic arterial infusion chemotherapy for hepatocellular carcinoma. Cancer Immunol Immunother. 2016;65:715–25.
35. Wang D, An G, Xie S, Yao Y, Feng G. The clinical and prognostic significance of CD14+HLA-DR−/low myeloid-derived suppressor cells in hepatocellular carcinoma patients receiving radiotherapy. Tumor Biol. 2016;37:10427–33. Springer Netherlands
36. Eggert T, Greten TF. Tumor regulation of the tissue environment in the liver. Pharmacol Ther. 2017;173:47–57.
37. Ji J, Eggert T, Budhu A, Forgues M, Takai A, Dang H, et al. Hepatic stellate cell and monocyte interaction contributes to poor prognosis in hepatocellular carcinoma. Hepatology. 2015;62:481–95.
38. Höchst B, Schildberg FA, Sauerborn P, Gäbel YA, Gevensleben H, Goltz D, et al. Activated human hepatic stellate cells induce myeloid derived suppressor cells from peripheral blood monocytes in a CD44-dependent fashion. J Hepatol. 2013;59:528–35.
39. Resheq YJ, Li K-K, Ward ST, Wilhelm A, Garg A, Curbishley SM, et al. Contact-dependent depletion of hydrogen peroxide by catalase is a novel mechanism of myeloid-derived suppressor cell induction operating in human hepatic stellate cells. J Immunol. 2015;194:2578–86. American Association of Immunologists
40. Yu M-C, Chen C-H, Liang X, Wang L, Gandhi CR, Fung JJ, et al. Inhibition of T-cell responses by hepatic stellate cells via B7-H1-mediated T-cell apoptosis in mice. Hepatology. 2004;40:1312–21. Wiley subscription services, Inc., A Wiley Company
41. Shevach EM. Regulatory T cells in autoimmmunity*. Annu Rev Immunol. 2000;18:423–49.
42. Speiser DE, Ho P-C, Verdeil G. Regulatory circuits of T cell function in cancer. Nat Rev Immunol. 2016;16:599–611.
43. Wiedemann GM, Knott MML, Vetter VK, Rapp M, Haubner S, Fesseler J, et al. Cancer cell-derived IL-1α induces CCL22 and the recruitment of regulatory T cells. Oncoimmunology. 2016;5:e1175794.
44. Ormandy LA, Hillemann T, Wedemeyer H, Manns MP, Greten TF, Korangy F. Increased populations of regulatory T cells in peripheral blood of patients with hepatocellular carcinoma. Cancer Res. 2005;65:2457–64.
45. Yang XH, Yamagiwa S, Ichida T, Matsuda Y, Sugahara S, Watanabe H, et al. Increase of CD4+ CD25+ regulatory T-cells in the liver of patients with hepatocellular carcinoma. J Hepatol. 2006;45:254–62.
46. Zhou J, Ding T, Pan W, Zhu L-Y, Li L, Zheng L. Increased intratumoral regulatory T cells are related to intratumoral macrophages and poor prognosis in hepatocellular carcinoma patients. Int J Cancer. 2009;125:1640–8.
47. Fu J, Xu D, Liu Z, Shi M, Zhao P, Fu B, et al. Increased regulatory T cells correlate with CD8 T-cell impairment and poor survival in hepatocellular carcinoma patients. Gastroenterology. 2007;132:2328–39.

48. Gao Q, Qiu SJ, Fan J, Zhou J, Wang XY, Xiao YS, et al. Intratumoral balance of regulatory and cytotoxic T cells is associated with prognosis of hepatocellular carcinoma after resection. J Clin Oncol. 2007;25:2586–93.
49. Kalathil S, Lugade AA, Miller A, Iyer R, Thanavala Y. Higher frequencies of GARP+CTLA-4+Foxp3+ T regulatory cells and myeloid-derived suppressor cells in hepatocellular carcinoma patients are associated with impaired T-cell functionality. Cancer Res. 2013;73:2435–44.
50. Greten TF, Ormandy LA, Fikuart A, Höchst B, Henschen S, Hörning M, et al. Low-dose cyclophosphamide treatment impairs regulatory T cells and unmasks AFP-specific CD4+ T-cell responses in patients with advanced HCC. J Immunother. 2010;33:211–8.
51. Motoyoshi Y, Kaminoda K, Saitoh O, Hamasaki K, Nakao K, Ishii N, et al. Different mechanisms for anti-tumor effects of low- and high-dose cyclophosphamide. Oncol Rep. 2006;16:141–6.
52. Kalathil SG, Lugade AA, Miller A, Iyer R, Thanavala Y. PD-1(+) and Foxp3(+) T cell reduction correlates with survival of HCC patients after sorafenib therapy. JCI Insight. 2016;1(11):pii: e86182.
53. Yang Z-Q, Yang Z-Y, Zhang L-D, Ping-Bie WS-G, Ma K-S, et al. Increased liver-infiltrating CD8+FoxP3+ regulatory T cells are associated with tumor stage in hepatocellular carcinoma patients. Hum Immunol. 2010;71:1180–6.
54. Ju C, Tacke F. Hepatic macrophages in homeostasis and liver diseases: from pathogenesis to novel therapeutic strategies. Cell Mol Immunol. 2016;13:316–27.
55. Tacke F, Zimmermann HW. Macrophage heterogeneity in liver injury and fibrosis. J Hepatol. 2014;60:1090–6.
56. Heymann F, Peusquens J, Ludwig-Portugall I, Kohlhepp M, Ergen C, Niemietz P, et al. Liver inflammation abrogates immunological tolerance induced by Kupffer cells. Hepatology. 2015;62:279–91.
57. Wu K, Kryczek I, Chen L, Zou W, Welling TH. Kupffer cell suppression of CD8+ T cells in human hepatocellular carcinoma is mediated by B7-H1/programmed death-1 interactions. Cancer Res. 2009;69:8067–75.
58. Zhu XD, Zhang JB, Zhuang PY, Zhu HG, Zhang W, Xiong YQ, et al. High expression of macrophage colony-stimulating factor in peritumoral liver tissue is associated with poor survival after curative resection of hepatocellular carcinoma. J Clin Oncol. 2008;26:2707–16. 2008 ed.
59. Budhu A, Forgues M, Ye Q-H, Jia H-L, He P, Zanetti KA, et al. Prediction of venous metastases, recurrence, and prognosis in hepatocellular carcinoma based on a unique immune response signature of the liver microenvironment. Cancer Cell. 2006;10:99–111.
60. Xiao X, Lao X-M, Chen M-M, Liu R-X, Wei Y, Ouyang F-Z, et al. PD-1hi identifies a novel regulatory B-cell population in human hepatoma that promotes disease progression. Cancer Discov. 2016;6:546–59.
61. Han Y, Chen Z, Yang Y, Jiang Z, Gu Y, Liu Y, et al. Human CD14+ CTLA-4+ regulatory dendritic cells suppress T-cell response by cytotoxic T-lymphocyte antigen-4-dependent IL-10 and indoleamine-2,3-dioxygenase production in hepatocellular carcinoma. Hepatology. 2014;59:567–79.
62. Zou W, Restifo NP. T(H)17 cells in tumour immunity and immunotherapy. Nat Rev Immunol. 2010;10:248–56. 2010 ed.
63. Zhao F, Hoechst B, Gamrekelashvili J, Ormandy LA, Voigtländer T, Wedemeyer H, et al. Human CCR4+CCR6+Th17 cells suppress autologous CD8+ T cell responses. J Immunol. 2012;188:6055–62.
64. Kaplan MH, Hufford MM, Olson MR. The development and in vivo function of T helper 9 cells. Nat Rev Immunol. 2015;15:295–307.
65. Tan H, Wang S, Zhao L. A tumour-promoting role of Th9 cells in hepatocellular carcinoma through CCL20 and STAT3 pathways. Clin Exp Pharmacol Physiol. 2017;44:213–21.
66. Quail DF, Joyce JA. Microenvironmental regulation of tumor progression and metastasis. Nat Med. 2013;19:1423–37.

67. Brandau S, Dumitru CA, Lang S. Protumor and antitumor functions of neutrophil granulocytes. Semin Immunopathol. 2013;35:163–76. Springer-Verlag
68. Zhou S-L, Zhou Z-J, Hu Z-Q, Huang X-W, Wang Z, Chen E-B, et al. Tumor-associated neutrophils recruit macrophages and T-regulatory cells to promote progression of hepatocellular carcinoma and resistance to Sorafenib. Gastroenterology. 2016;150:1646–1658.e17.
69. Xing F, Saidou J, Watabe K. Cancer associated fibroblasts (CAFs) in tumor microenvironment. Front Biosci. 2010;15:166–79. (Landmark Ed)
70. Deng Y, Cheng J, Fu B, Liu W, Chen G, Zhang Q, et al. Hepatic carcinoma-associated fibroblasts enhance immune suppression by facilitating the generation of myeloid-derived suppressor cells. Oncogene. 2016;36(8):1090–101.
71. De Palma M, Venneri MA, Galli R, Sergi Sergi L, Politi LS, Sampaolesi M, et al. Tie2 identifies a hematopoietic lineage of proangiogenic monocytes required for tumor vessel formation and a mesenchymal population of pericyte progenitors. Cancer Cell. 2005;8:211–26.
72. Murdoch C, Tazzyman S, Webster S, Lewis CE. Expression of tie-2 by human monocytes and their responses to angiopoietin-2. J Immunol. 2007;178:7405–11.
73. Venneri MA, De Palma M, Ponzoni M, Pucci F, Scielzo C, Zonari E, et al. Identification of proangiogenic TIE2-expressing monocytes (TEMs) in human peripheral blood and cancer. Blood. 2007;109:5276–85. American Society of Hematology
74. Matsubara T, Kanto T, Kuroda S, Yoshio S, Higashitani K, Kakita N, et al. TIE2-expressing monocytes as a diagnostic marker for hepatocellular carcinoma correlates with angiogenesis. Hepatology. 2013;57:1416–25. Wiley Subscription Services, Inc., A Wiley Company
75. Cabrera R, Tu Z, Xu Y, Firpi RJ, Rosen HR, Liu C, et al. An immunomodulatory role for CD4(+)CD25(+) regulatory T lymphocytes in hepatitis C virus infection. Hepatology. 2004;40:1062–71.
76. Cabrera R, Ararat M, Cao M, Xu Y, Wasserfall C, Atkinson MA, et al. Hepatocellular carcinoma immunopathogenesis: clinical evidence for global T cell defects and an immunomodulatory role for soluble CD25 (sCD25). Dig Dis Sci. 2010;55:484–95. 2009 ed.
77. Cabrera R, Ararat M, Eksioglu EA, Cao M, Xu Y, Wasserfall C, et al. Influence of serum and soluble CD25 (sCD25) on regulatory and effector T-cell function in hepatocellular carcinoma. Scand J Immunol. 2010;72:293–301. 2010 ed.
78. Cariani E, Pilli M, Zerbini A, Rota C, Olivani A, Pelosi G, et al. Immunological and molecular correlates of disease recurrence after liver resection for hepatocellular carcinoma. PLoS One. 2012;7:e32493.
79. Zeng Z, Shi F, Zhou L, Zhang M-N, Chen Y, Chang X-J, et al. Upregulation of circulating PD-L1/PD-1 is associated with poor post-cryoablation prognosis in patients with HBV-related hepatocellular carcinoma. Luk J, editor. PLoS ONE. 2011;6:e23621.
80. Wang B-J. Immunostaining of PD-1/PD-ls in liver tissues of patients with hepatitis and hepatocellular carcinoma. World J Gastroenterol. 2011;17:3322–8.
81. Gao Q, Wang XY, Qiu SJ, Yamato I, Sho M, Nakajima Y, et al. Overexpression of PD-L1 significantly associates with tumor aggressiveness and postoperative recurrence in human hepatocellular carcinoma. Clin Cancer Res. 2009;15:971–9. 2009 ed.
82. Semaan A, Dietrich D, Bergheim D, Dietrich J, Kalff JC, Branchi V, et al. CXCL12 expression and PD-L1 expression serve as prognostic biomarkers in HCC and are induced by hypoxia. Virchows Arch. 2016;470:185–96. Springer Berlin Heidelberg
83. Pardee AD, Shi J, Butterfield LH. Tumor-derived -fetoprotein impairs the differentiation and T cell stimulatory activity of human dendritic cells. J Immunol. 2014;193:5723–32.
84. Bricard G, Cesson V, Devevre E, Bouzourene H, Barbey C, Rufer N, et al. Enrichment of human CD4+ V(alpha)24/Vbeta11 invariant NKT cells in intrahepatic malignant tumors. J Immunol. 2009;182:5140–51.

Chapter 9
Impact of Cytokines in Hepatocellular Carcinoma Initiation and Progression

Yeni Ait-Ahmed and Fouad Lafdil

Over the past several decades, numerous studies have shown that inflammatory diseases and infections trigger or promote the development and progression of many types of cancers [65], including hepatocellular carcinoma (HCC) which occurs in most cases at late stages of chronic liver disease associated with viral hepatitis B and C infection, metabolic disorders, and alcohol heavy consumption [41].

Chronic liver diseases, whatever their etiologies, are often associated with a sustained inflammatory response leading to repeated injury, fibrosis and at late stages, to cirrhosis. HCC arises in the setting of cirrhotic livers in 80 to 90% of cases and progresses in an inflammatory context. Despite significant progress in HCC diagnosis and improvement of the curative strategies, its incidence is still increasing in western countries and the prognosis of patients with advanced HCC remains in general very poor. Recurrence and non-response to the current anti-cancer treatment occur frequently. Diverse immune cell types associated with the release of a large spectrum of inflammatory cytokines appeared to be a key component in HCC emergence, progression and in therapeutic failures. Many factors produced by infiltrating immune cells such as chemokines, growth factors, cytokines and proangiogenic factors contribute to the promotion of cell survival, proliferation, epithelial-mesenchymal transition and genomic DNA instability [55].

Y. Ait-Ahmed
Université Paris-Est, Faculté des Sciences et Technologies, UMR-S955, Créteil F-94000, France

Laboratory of Liver Diseases, National Institute on Alcohol Abuse and Alcoholism, National Institutes of Health, Bethesda, MD, USA

F. Lafdil (✉)
Université Paris-Est, Faculté des Sciences et Technologies, UMR-S955, Créteil F-94000, France

INSERM, U955, Créteil F-94000, France

Institut Universitaire de France (IUF), Paris F-75231 Cedex 05, France
e-mail: fouad.lafdil@inserm.fr

T.F. Greten (ed.), *Immunotherapy of Hepatocellular Carcinoma*,
DOI 10.1007/978-3-319-64958-0_9

Thus, a better characterization of the underlying molecular and cellular mechanisms by which HCC development and resistance occur may open new insights for the development of more effective anticancer therapies. In addition to curative strategies for HCC, it is of interest to identify and block the immune cell types and their associated cytokines susceptible to trigger tumor initiation and progression.

9.1 Cytokines in Chronic Liver Diseases: A Risk Factor for HCC Initiation

9.1.1 Chronic Alcohol Consumption is a Risk Factor for HCC Emergence

Chronic alcohol consumption is associated with hepatic inflammation leading to cirrhosis development, and constitute a risk factor for HCC initiation. Chronic liver diseases are mainly due to recurrent and excessive liver inflammatory processes, as observed in alcoholic liver disease (ALD). ALD ranks among the major causes of morbidity and mortality worldwide, with a mortality rate in the USA and in Western Europe estimated to be approximately 5–6%. In USA, ALD is responsible for up to 100,000 deaths per year. ALD can present as steatosis (fatty liver, i.e. accumulation of triglycerides in hepatocytes), the prevalent lesion found in excessive drinkers that is now recognized as harbinger of worse disease to follow when liver insult is sustained. Indeed, steatosis may progress towards alcoholic steatohepatitis (ASH), when accompanied with liver inflammation and hepatocyte injury, that promotes liver fibrogenesis with a 20% risk of cirrhosis after 10–20 years. Severe alcoholic hepatitis (AH) is a specific clinical form characterized by a prolonged and intense **inflammatory reaction** despite alcohol withdrawal, and associated with a spontaneous 50% mortality rate after 6 months. Current management of steatosis and mild to moderate forms of AH relies upon abstinence. In severe AH, corticosteroids reduce the mortality rate to 15–20% after 6 months. Nevertheless, outcome after 1 year remains grim with survival rates ranging between 50 to 60%. Overall, these figures underscore the urgent need for **novel therapeutic approaches targeting inflammation** in the management of ALD.

9.1.1.1 Role of Innate Immune Cytokines

Activation of hepatic innate immune cells is the first step that triggers inflammation in alcoholic patients. Indeed, dysregulated cytokine signaling, particularly of those released by the resident macrophages of the liver (Kupffer cells), plays a pivotal role in the pathogenesis of ALD. In particular, several clinical and experimental studies have shown that overproduction of **TNF-α** by activated Kupffer cells is central to the inflammatory process associated with ALD [95, 121, 126]. The mechanism leading to increased **TNF-α** production in response to ethanol involves enhanced intra-hepatic oxidative stress and altered gut permeability, thereby allowing enhanced translocation of endotoxin (LPS) into the portal blood, and activation of Kupffer cells following binding of LPS to its receptor Toll Like Receptor 4 (TLR4). TNF-α [141] induces hepatocyte cell death and inflammatory cell infiltration [12]. Furthermore, liver regeneration has also been shown to be impaired in ALD [60]. In addition, clinical treatments of patients with severe AH based on TNF-α neutralization with pentoxifilin (PTX) [1] or monoconal antibodies like infliximab [104] or etanercept [13] have been shown to prevent inflammation but were associated with severe side effects including a higher susceptibility to infection leading to increased mortality rate. In addition, above and beyond its detrimental role in liver inflammation, TNF-α is not only critical for the host defence, but it also induces IL-6 synthesis to initiate hepatocyte proliferation and liver regeneration. IL-6 and TNF-α are two cytokines mainly produced by Kupffer cells in the liver and markedly induced after partial hepatectomy. TNF-α is a major regulator of the initiation of liver regeneration. It is known that IL-6 and TNF-α can stimulate hepatocyte proliferation by activating intracellular signalling pathways such as signal transducer and activator of transcription 3 (STAT-3) and CCAAT/enhancer-binding protein B (C/EBP). Altogether, these data point out the importance of controlling the balance between the inflammatory immune response required for pathogen elimination and liver regeneration, and the exacerbated inflammatory processes leading to hepatocyte cell death.

The molecular mechanisms associated with Kupffer cell activation are linked to acquisition of an **M1 phenotype** characterized by the production of a storm of inflammatory cytokines including TNF-α, IL-6, IL-12 and IFN-γ, which supports resistance to extracellular bacterial infection. However, overwhelming production of those cytokines by Kupffer cells is responsible for the development of AH. Contrastingly, **M2-polarized macrophages** are defined by production of IL-10, IL-4, and IL-13. Although those macrophages cannot control bacterial infection, they are critical for tempering the triggered inflammatory process, and in promoting tissue repair. And recently an **atypical M2 profile** has been reported that combines M1 and M2 characteristics [11] producing IL-6, TGF-β and the chemokine CXCL8 (also known as IL-8) susceptible to promote liver fibrosis.

Dendritic cells (DCs) are professional antigen presenting cells. They have the unique capacity to catch, process and load all kinds of antigens and prime effectors immune cells namely $CD4^+$ and $CD8^+$ T cells. Basically, two types of DCs are described. The first DC type conventional DCs respond to lipopolysaccharide and lipoteichoic acid via TLR4 and TLR2, respectively, and produce TNF-α, IL-6, IL-12. The second DC type known as plasmacitoid DCs respond to TLR7 and TLR9 activation by producing IFN-α [102]. Impaired DC functions highly contribute to tumor escape from immune-surveillance in patients with cancer [44].

9.1.1.2 Impact of Adaptive Immune Response

Indeed, in addition to the crucial role of macrophages, increasing evidence also points out the crucial role of T lymphocytes in mediating hepatitis in ALD [8, 17, 77]. The decrease in peripheral lymphocyte number is associated with an increase in the ratio of T helper cells to suppressor cells in the liver. Today, four major distinct $CD4^+$ T cell subtypes have been described: the Th1, Th2, T regulatory (Treg) and more recently, the Th17 phenotype.

Th1 cells that mainly produce IFN-γ, mediate immune response against intracellular pathogens, and are also involved in some autoimmune diseases [99, 107].

Th2 cells that produce principally IL-4, IL-10 and IL-13 are involved in host defence against extracellular parasites [99, 107] and suppress Th1 cell proliferation [38].

Th17 cells defined as producer of IL-17, IL-21 and IL-22, play a major role in immune response against bacteria and fungi and participate also to the induction of several autoimmune diseases [133], but could also protect hepatocytes in acute hepatitis through IL-22 production [142]. Recently, the deleterious role of T helper lymphocytes secreting IL-17 (Th17 cells) in recruiting neutrophils has been reported in ALD [88]. In addition, persistent IL-17 production has been identified in numerous other chronic liver diseases with deleterious functions leading to cirrhosis and HCC development [52, 84]. These findings strongly support the potent role of T cells in the progression of AH. Indeed, T helper differentiation into a specific phenotype is mainly controlled by innate immune cells that in turn could respond to the variety of produced cytokines by those differentiated T cells.

Treg cells regulate immune response by maintaining the self-tolerance and are beneficial for treating autoimmune diseases [118]. First described as suppressive T cells, [118] Treg lymphocytes are involved in immunosuppression and mainly contribute to tumor immune escape. $CD4^+$ $CD25^{high}$ $FoxP3^+$ Treg cells are induced by several microenvironmental factors including IL-10, TGF-β and VEGF which are overexpressed in HCC [10, 50, 140]. However, studies have reported a negative correlation between an increase in Treg infiltrating cells and clinical outcome in HCC patients [58]. In addition, it has been shown that in many types of liver disorders including chronic viral hepatitis, liver cirrhosis and HCC, Treg cell number increase favored HCC appearance and growth [74]. IL-10 mainly produced by Treg is the most studied anti-inflammatory cytokine regarding HCC. It has been shown that IL-10 is overexpressed in patients with HCC with less optimistic prognosis compared [10, 21]. Consistent with the previous studies, these reports strongly suggest that through IL-10 production, Treg lymphocytes promote HCC progression.

9.1.1.3 Inflammation-Associated Reactive Oxygen and Nitrogen Species (ROS and RNS)

Notable discoveries in mechanisms involved in ALD demonstrated the critical role of Kupffer cells in mediating AH through TNF-α overproduction, and led scientists to propose therapeutic strategies neutralizing TNF-α-mediated inflammation. In association with TNF-α, over-production of IL-6 was pointed out as driving factor of liver carcinogenesis [106]. The major mechanism that has been highlighted is the IL-6-induced reactive oxygen species (ROS) production and epigenetic changes triggering HCC development [123].

Due to ethanol oxidization by the cytochrome CYP2E1, acetaldehyde and reactive oxygen species (ROS) accumulate in the liver. This ROS accumulation promotes lipid peroxidation, DNA damage, chromosome instability and epigenetic disturbance. In an inflammatory context, epithelial and immune cell activation induce the production of reactive oxygen and nitrogen species (RONS) by NADPH oxidase, and nitric oxide synthase (NOS). Studies on chronic inflammatory diseases including inflammatory bowel diseases (IBD) and Helicobacter pylori-induced gastritis have reported increased level of RONS, suggesting a link between RONS production and cancer risk [111, 116]. RONS production induces cell damages including oxidative stress, lipids, proteins and DNA abnormalities through 8-oxodG and 8-nitrodeoxyguanosine accumulation [101] and therefore promote tumor initiation and malignancy. The discovery of RONS-induced DNA damages in chronic inflammatory responses including hepatitis is consistent with the involvement of RONS in diseases characterized by a higher cancer risk [101]. Furthermore, 8-oxodG and 8-nitrodeoxyguanine reactivity plays an important role in hepatitis C virus-induced chronic hepatitis [61]. All together these observations enhance the link between inflammation-induced RONS and carcinogenesis. Therapeutical use of antioxidants (e.g., *S*-adenosyl-L-methionine, polyunsaturated phosphatidylcholine) to restore alcohol-induced methionine and oxidative balance disruption, has shown promising effects but still needs to be further studied [115].

9.1.2 Cytokines in Fibrosis and Increased Risk of HCC Initiation

Tissue damage due to sustained inflammation leads in most cases to fibrosis development. Liver fibrosis is caused by a large variety of chronic liver diseases and represents an important cause of mortality in the world. The immune system protects the host from foreign pathogens without disrupting tolerance toward self-antigens but during fibrogenesis, inflammation contribute to the deposition and accumulation of collagen leading to an important modification of the physiological liver architecture.

Hepatic stellate cells represent the major cell population responsible for increased deposition of extracellular matrix proteins including collagen molecules. Collagens can also be produced to a lesser extent by other cell types including progenitor cells, portal fibroblasts, and cholangiocytes. Many immune cells including Kupffer cells, natural killer cells and dendritic cells have been shown to participate to liver fibrogenesis by releasing pro-inflammatory cytokines. These cytokines such as IFN-α and IFN-β, IL-6 and IL-22, activate the JAK-STAT signaling pathways by binding to their respective receptors.

9.1.2.1 Antifibrotic Cytokines

Interferon type 1, 2 and 3 were identified as cytokines that in general inhibit liver fibrosis development. For instance, IFN-α treatment significantly reduces the hepatic fibrosis in mice by blocking collagen gene transcription via the interaction of p300 transcription factor and phosphorylated STAT1 [66]. Similarly, IFN-γ deficient mice are more susceptible to develop liver fibrosis induced by CCl_4 administration or under a 3,5-diethoxycarbonyl-1,4-dihydrocollidine (DDC) diet [67, 112]. The anti-fibrotic function of IFN-γ are more likely mediated through the induction of hepatic stellate cell-growth arrest and apoptosis [112].

It has been recently demonstrated that triple knockout mice for IL-10, IL-12/23 and IL-13Ra2 are more susceptible to many pathologies related to liver including S. mansoni-induced liver fibrosis model. Levels of liver enzymes, hepatosplenomegaly and ascites were increased, suggesting that IL-10, IL-12p40, and IL-13Rα2 contribute cooperatively to reduce liver fibrosis in this model of S. mansoni infected mice [97].

In the liver, IL-6 and IL-22 are mainly responsible for the activation of STAT3.

IL-6 knock-out mice seems more susceptible to liver injury and fibrosis after CCl_4 treatment [79]. Furthermore, the lack of gp130/STAT3-mediated signaling in hepatocytes leads to worsened DDC diet feeding related chronic cholestatic liver injury and fibrosis progression [109]. Similarly, hepatocyte-specific STAT3 knockout mice displays a higher degree of liver fibrosis compared with wild-type mice in various models of liver fibrosis induced by CCl_4 administration, feeding with a 3,5-diethoxycarbonyl-1,4-dihydrocollidine (DDC) diet [109], feeding with a choline-deficient, ethionine-supplemented (CDE) diet [80].

In hepatocytes, STAT5 activation is mainly induced by growth hormone (GH). Using the hepatocyte-specific STAT5 knockout mice developed in Dr. Lothar Hennighausen's laboratory [26], STAT5 loss in hepatocytes has been shown to promote increased TGF-β levels and enhanced STAT3 activity induced by GH in the liver after CCl_4 administration [6, 62]. Moreover, STAT5 deletion in the liver promoted hepatic tumorigenesis induced by CCl_4 injection in wild-type mice [62] and was responsible for the development of spontaneous liver cancer in liver-specific glucocorticoid receptor knockout mice [100] or in GH transgenic mice [43]. Although the effects of STAT5 in hepatocytes have been widely investigated, little is known about the potential functions of STAT5 in the fibrogenic hepatic stellate cells (HSC).

9.1.2.2 Pro-fibrotic Cytokines

It is also known that IFN-α/β and IL-12 can activate STAT4 in immune cells and promote inflammation. In several animal models, treatment with IL-12 has been shown to induce liver inflammation and reduce liver tumor growth [18, 57]. This inflammatory response is characterized by the activation of NK and NKT cells which in turn produce IFN-γ [124]. Via the activation of STAT4 in immune cells, IL-12 seems to act as a pro-inflammatory cytokine promoting fibrosis and liver injury.

Th2 cytokines such as IL-4 and IL-13 are considered to be pro-inflammatory. Studies have shown that administration of IL-13 inhibitors or IL-13 gene blockage results in a significant reduction of liver fibrosis in the S. mansoni infection model. In humans, a correlation has been established between elevated levels of IL-13 and liver fibrosis in patients with chronic HBV or HCV infection, suggesting that IL-13 promotes liver fibrosis in an infection dependent or independent context [135]. These pro-fibrogenic effects can be explained by the fact that IL-13 induces HSC activation and promotes the production of fibrotic proteins by HSCs in a STAT6 dependent manner. Indeed, STAT6 blockage with siRNA inhibits HSC activation in vitro [3, 122]. Moreover, STAT6-deficient mice present smaller amounts of collagen deposition in the liver compared with wild- type mice after infection with S. mansoni [71]. Like TGF-β, IL-4 is known to have pro-fibrotic properties as it contributes to HSC activation and collagen production [3, 69]. Furthermore, IL-4 expression levels are higher in fibrotic liver from S. mansoni-infected baboons [37]. Although the role of IL-13 in liver fibrosis is reported in the S. mansoni infection model, studies to come need to clarify to what extent STAT6 in HSC is implicated in liver fibrogenesis in patients with chronic liver diseases.

IL-6 is a major pro-regenerative factor and induces the acute phase in the liver by stimulating hepatocytes to produce acute phase proteins such as C-reactive protein, serum amyloid A and complement C3 [114]. Clinical studies showed that IL-6 hepatic expression is increased and positively correlated with the degree of liver fibrosis [32, 136]. As IL-6 receptors are widely expressed on all types of cells in the liver, it can explain how IL-6 may have distinct roles in all these types of cells by regulating positively and negatively liver fibrosis. It has been shown that IL-6 can directly promote HSC survival and proliferation resulting in enhanced liver fibrosis. Collectively, the major effect of IL-6 on liver fibrosis is the result of the balance between on the one hand the inhibitory effect through STAT3 activation in hepatocytes and the stimulatory effects enhancing HSC survival, which depend on liver fibrosis stage and etiology.

9.1.3 Influence of Cytokines in Liver Progenitor/Stem Cell Activation: A Potent Mechanism of HCC Initiation

Liver progenitor cell (LPC) proliferation is reported in ductular reaction, often observed, in cirrhotic livers, hepatitis B and C viral infections, alcoholic or non-alcoholic steatohepatitis. Their appearance is associated with increased incidence of HCC. An interest in LPC biology emerged because of their stem-cell-like capacities to promote liver regeneration and to generate liver cancer. LPCs can differentiate into mature hepatocytes and biliary cells. Their capacity to restore injured hepatic tissue has been well documented [36]. However, LPCs were also defined as precursors for HCC and described as potent Cancer Stem Cells (CSCs) when they undergo "transformation" and generate heterogeneous lineage of cancer cells [29, 73, 94, 117]. Many transcription factors such as NANOG, cMYC, KLF-4, OCT4, SOX2 are stemness markers which have been reported to be increased in cancers [131].

The signaling pathways identified in HCC are also observed in isolated liver CSCs (eg, Wnt, Notch, TGF-β, Hedgehog, and PI3K/AKT/mTOR [86, 87]. Liver CSCs can be identified based on the expression of several cell markers such as CD90, CD44, CD24, CD13, epithelial cell adhesion molecule (EpCAM), CD133 (prominin-1), and oval cell marker OV6 as well as Hoechst dye efflux or aldehyde dehydrogenase expression and activities [86, 87]. Among those markers, double positive CD133+ and EpCAM+ cells display higher expression of stem-cell related genes and appearance of drug-resistance to chemotherapeutics. CSCs can initiate tumor in xenograft transplantation experiments. Moreover, the high capacity of resistance of CSC to sorafenib therapy suggests that CSCs could contribute to the poor prognosis [54] and participate to HCC recurrence. Several lines of evidence suggest a potential role of inflammatory microenvironment in CSC-initiation and progression towards HCC.

Recently, a correlation between IGF-1R and the expression of stemness markers in HBV-related HCC has been reported and suggests that inflammatory cytokines are involved in CSC development. The hepatic microenvironment is markedly disrupted in chronic liver diseases and characterized by infiltration of lymphocytes, activation of stellate cells and expansion of hepatic progenitor cells. One of the main axis involved in liver inflammation is IL-6/STAT3 signaling that in collaboration with TGF-β potentially promotes CSC survival and proliferation in the liver [98, 125].

9.2 Mechanisms of Cytokine Contribution to Tumor Growth

9.2.1 Role of Inflammation Related micro-RNA in HCC Development

In addition to its ability to modulate liver immune response, alcohol can also lead to epigenetic changes in inflammatory-associated genes via the multiple mechanisms [27]. These include (i) DNA-methyl transferases increasing methylation on gene promoters, (ii) an alteration of the physiological interaction between the transcriptional proteins to the DNA due to inappropriate methylation, acetylation phosphorylation and/or ubiquitination, and (iii) more recently, a transcriptional regulation mediated by micro-RNAs (miRNA) [102]. Epigenetic regulation of DNA methylation, phosphorylation, and ubiquitination by alcohol has been extensively reviewed in many previous articles. Here we mainly discuss the role of miRNAs in pathogenesis of HCC.

MiRNA are single-stranded non-coding RNAs composed of 20 nucleotides approximately. They are mostly responsible for the post-transcriptional epigenetic regulation of targeted gene expression. The interest for the miRNA raised when evidence of aberrant expression of several miRNAs was reported in many types of cancers [15]. Many pathways such as p53, RAS/MAPK, PI3K/ AKT/mTOR, WNT/ β-catenin, and TGF-β are involved in HCC development. Abnormal expression of some miRNA has been observed in HCC compared to normal liver tissue [105]. It has been shown that miRNA-199a and miRNA-122 are highly expressed in healthy liver. Interestingly, the expression of these two miRNAs is markedly disrupted in HCC [63]. MiR-199 has been shown to stop cell cycle at G1 phase. A correlation has been reported between the downregulation of miR-199a (a member of miR-199 family) and increased recurrence rate with reduced laps before recurrence of HCC [68].

MiR-122 is only expressed in adult normal liver and seems to be a key factor in the regulation of hepatocyte differentiation by inhibiting genes not exclusive to the liver [139] which makes it a particular miRNA in liver physiopathology. Consistent with these findings, in up to 70% of HCC, miR-122 is downregulated indicating that this miRNA should have an antitumor activity. Furthermore, miR-122 is known to promote apoptosis, block the tumor cell cycle, reduce in vivo cancer cell malignancy and increase efficacy of drugs such as Sorafenib and also doxorubicin by inhibiting p53 activity [5, 40]. Interestingly, in liver cancer patients, miR-122 loss is correlated with the development of metastasis and a reduced period before recurrence [25, 127]. Thanks to a miR-122 KO mouse model, the role of this miR is now better defined [64, 128]. MiR-122KO developed chronic liver inflammation, fibrosis and HCC like spontaneous tumors comforting the antitumor potential of miR-122. Indeed, miR122 targets CULT-1 and reduces its activity which explain the undifferentiated phenotype of HCC cells. Similar to miR-199, miR-122 inhibits cyclin G1 leading to an upregulation of p53 which is increased in HCC [51]. The link between miRNA and the inflammatory response seems very strong suggesting that some cytokines could be involved in miRNA regulation. This mechanism by which cytokines could induce some miRNA targeting antitumor genes and thus promote tumor growth seems to be a very promising axis to explore in carcinogenesis.

In a study, up to 80% of HCC analyses showed a significant increase of miR-221 expression. This upregulation of miR-221 leads to increased tumor growth and cancer cell proliferation [47, 96]. Consistent with these observations, in transgenic mice overexpressing miR-221 in the liver, higher HCC tumorigenicity was reported and could be inhibited by administrating anti-miR-221 nucleotides, called antagomiR [16].

9.2.2 Cytokine-Induced Oncogenic Intracellular Pathways

Raf/MAPK/ERK signaling pathway is involved in cell growth and differentiation. The extracellular signal is translated from tyrosine kinase receptors including VEGFR, IGFR, PDGFR, EGFR and MET, triggering a cascade of intracellular phosphorylations [4]. RAS, a GTPase protein, and Raf, a serine/threonine kinase regulate the signal transduction in this pathway [75]. A study has shown that in HCC Raf kinase inhibitor is down-regulated leading to an over-activity of the Raf/MAPK/ERK pathway [85]. New therapeutic approaches including Sorafenib aimed to target and inhibit Raf kinase, and consequently to limit tumor growth [137].

PI3K/Akt/mTOR like the Raf/MAPK/ERK signaling pathway, controls proliferation, growth, motility and cell survival. HCC patients present an over-activation of this pathway. Indeed, it has been reported that in over 40% of HCC patients, Akt signaling and mTOR effector (p70s6k) were activated leading to increased cell survival and growth through an inhibition of TGF-β induced apoptosis [20]. These observations highlighted this signaling pathway as a potential target for therapeutic perspectives. Some strategies have been developed to block this pathway such as PI-103 inhibiting the phosphoinositide 3 Kinase (PI3K) and mTOR activation. These treatments showed efficacy in blocking Raf/MAP/ERK and PI3K/Akt/mTOR pathways leading to the reduction of EGF-induced proliferation of tumor cells [48].

Wnt/β-catenin targets many processes including cell determination, stemness but also intercellular adhesion by interacting with E-cadherin and proliferative signal transmission through β-catenin activity [110]. Aberrant Beta-catenin activation is found in almost 40% of human HCC. B-catenin degradation is regulated by Adenomatous Polyposis Coli (APC) protein [22, 23]. Growth factors from the extracellular microenvironment bind to the Frizzled (Fzd) receptors expressed on the cell surface and activate this pathway. In murine and human HCC, an abnormal activity of this pathway has been reported [30, 56]. In absence of Wnt, the destruction complex formed by AXIN1, adenomatous polyposis coli (APC), glycogen synthase kinase-3β (GSK-3β), and casein kinase 1 (CK1) proteins drive the proteolysis of β-catenin through the ubiquitin/proteasome mechanism by phosphorylating the protein. Another protein has been reported to be increased in HCC; PRC1 controls cytoskeleton organization and increase Wnt signaling by contributing to the sequestration of the complex at the membrane, promoting tumorigenesis and metastasis development [19]. The role of Wnt/β-catenin in tumor growth is an attractive field to explore for paving the way to new therapeutic options. Indeed, antibody based therapies have already been developed. Blocking the β-catenin signaling reduced HCC tumor growth and increased apoptosis through the administration of anti-Wnt-1 antibodies [134].

NF-κB plays a central role in liver injury, fibrosis and HCC development [91]. Its activation in macrophages lead to a large production of cytokines shaping an inflammatory tumor microenvironment of HCC [72]. In a DEN induced HCC murine model, Kupffer cell and hepatocyte specific blockade of IKK-β which is a major activator of NF-κB, leads to decrease tumor size and reduced the production of inflammatory cytokines including TNF-α and IL-6. However, an increase of hepatotumorigenesis was reported with a deletion of IKK-β only in hepatocytes [92]. These paradoxical results highlight the double-edged sword role and complexity of NF-κB signaling but clearly show the key role played by immune cells in shaping a favorable pro-tumor microenvironment.

9.2.3 Cytokine Gene Polymorphisms Contribute to Altered Immune Response

In addition to the environmental factors responsible for cytokine release during chronic liver diseases, alteration in cytokine or cytokine receptor gene expressions can occur and chronically dysregulate the inflammatory response leading to cancer development. Such alteration results from single nucleotide polymorphisms (SNPs) in coding or non-coding regions of the genes. Several cytokine gene polymorphisms have been recently reported, including IL-1β [34], resulting in increased cytokine release. Furthermore, genetic polymorphisms of IL-6 are associated with fibrosis progression in chronic HCV infected patients [28]. Polymorphisms were identified in virtually all other cytokines such as TNF-α, IL-6, IL-10, TGF-β1 and IFN-γ [33].

9.3 Cytokines in HCC Progression with Metastasis

Tumor microenvironment is shaped by myeloid and lymphoid cells including tumor infiltrating lymphocytes (TILs) responsible for the control of tumor growth (Fig. 9.1). According to their phenotypes myeloid and lymphoid cells will inhibit or promote tumor growth. Myeloid cells basically play a major role in the immune response against tumor by recognizing these tumor antigens and generating humoral and cellular specific immune responses. However, their ability in tumor-associated

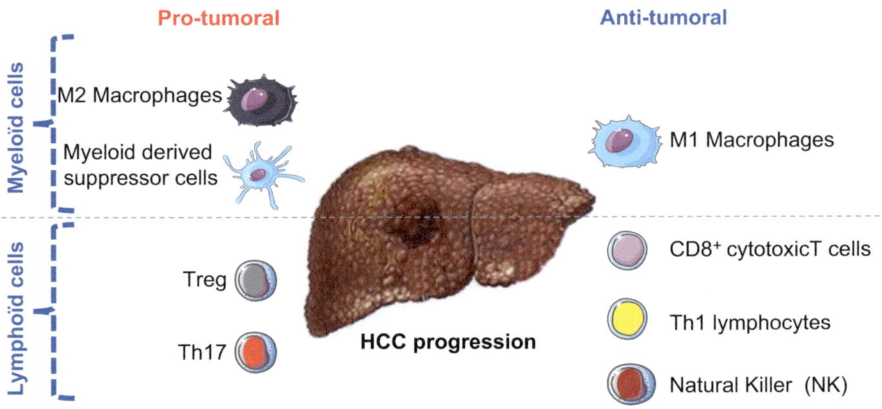

Fig. 9.1 Immune cell microenvironment of HCC. The HCC microenvironment is composed of pro-tumoral immune cells including M2 macrophages, myeloid derived supressor cells, Treg and Th17 lymphocytes, and anti-tumoral cells gathering M1 macrophages, cytotoxic CD8 T cells, Th1 and NK cells

antigen recognition is often altered and lead to pro-tumoral properties of those cells. Among lymphoid cells, two types of TILs can be distinguished: anti-tumoral effector cells such as $CD8^+$ lymphocytes which are associated with a better prognosis when they are highly present in the tumor, that are opposed to pro-tumoral cells such as regulatory T cells (Treg) which are associated with a poor prognosis.

9.3.1 Myeloid Immune Response in HCC Progression

Tumor Associated Macrophages (TAMs) also play a key regulatory role in tumor-related inflammation and angiogenesis. TAMs are also involved in tumor relapse by facilitating tumor regrowth, revascularization, and spread after anti-cancer therapies. TAMs are associated to tumor growth through the production of growth factors such as EGF, VEGF and bFGF. They contribute to the invasiveness of tumor cells and metastasis by favoring extracellular matrix remodeling via the release of metalloproteases 2 and 9 (MMP2 and MMP9). They also contribute to vascularize the tumor by increasing angiogenesis and lymphangiogenesis via MMP9, VEGF and PDGF synthesis [45].

Tumor-associated neutrophils (TAN) similarly to TAMs, have been described [93] CXCL8 chemokine production by tumoral cells in HCC are responsible for the chemotaxis of neutrophils in the stroma surrounding the nodules [83]. More recently, an analysis of 919 HCC identified an overexpression of the CXCL5 chemokine that correlated with an increase in neutrophil-infiltrating cells in the liver and a poor prognosis of the diseases [144]. Those recruited neutrophils favors tumoral progression in part by increase in ROS production (as mentioned earlier in this chapter)

[55]. Interestingly, neutrophil-derived ROS was associated with mutations and DNA damage [53] and activation of proteolytic enzymes including MMP-2, 7, 8, 9 and inactivation of the Tissue inhibitor metalloprotease-1 (TIMP-1) which consequently favour tumor invasiveness [31].

Myeloid Derived-Suppressor Cells (MDSCs) represent a heterogeneous population of cells sharing similarities with TAMs and TANs. They are often observed in HCC and their presence is associated with a poor prognosis. This population of cells is basically composed of main sub-types: monocytic MDSCs and granulocytic MDSCs. Under certain conditions they can adopt several phenotypes that control their ability to promote or restrain tumor progression. For instance, in hypoxic conditions or in presence of tumor -derived factions, MDSC can differentiate into immunosuppressive TAMs [24]. Furthermore studies reported in vitro their capacity to differentiate in a macrophage, DC or granulocyte phenotype [103]. However, in general, MDSCs are described as suppressor of T cell activation and therefore can alter T-cell mediated anti-tumor function and favour tumor progression [130].

9.3.2 Lymphoid Immune Response in HCC Progression

9.3.2.1 Infiltrating $CD8^+$ T Cells and Their Associated Cytokines

$CD8^+$ T cells are major actors in antitumor immunity through their antigen specific cytotoxicity capacities targeting tumor antigens. These latter are ingested by host antigen presenting cell such as dendritic cells and processed into peptides which are presented via class I and class II MHC molecules respectively to $CD8^+$ and $CD4^+$T cells. In many cancer including colorectal and ovarian cancers, an increased number of tumor infiltrating $CD8^+$ T lymphocytes (TIL) predicts a favorable prognosis. Regarding HCC, a correlation has also been reported between the presence of TIL and patient prognosis [46]. Indeed, the penetration of $CD8^+$ T cells is correlated to an improved recurrence-free survival after liver resection [59]. These beneficial effects are explained by the inflammatory microenvironment generated by $CD8^+$ effector T cells within the tumor leading to the establishment of an anti-tumor response. Studies have shown in murine models that through IL-12 stimulation, $CD8^+$ T cells were activated which induce IFN-γ release leading to increased hepatoma cell apoptosis [76].

Recent findings [39] have highlighted $CD8^+$ T specific responses targeting tumor-associated antigens (TAA) in HCC. It has been shown that TAA-specific $CD8^+$ T cell immune response was visible in more than 1 out of 2 HCC patients and already detectable in early stages of the disease. Consistent with the correlation between improved progression-free survival TAA-specific $CD8^+$ T responses these results comfort the major role played by these cells in anti-tumor immunity.

However, in some patients with HCC, impaired functions of $CD8^+$ T cells have been reported [49]. Indeed, tumors develop mechanisms to escape to immune surveillance; one of them is the up-regulation of the ligand for PD-1 (PD-L1) responsible for addressing an inhibitory signal to PD-1 expressing cells namely $CD8^+$ and $CD4^+$ T cells [42]. This PD1/PD-L1 interaction leads to T cell inactivation and consequently, to the inhibition of their anti-tumor function and ultimately to the promotion of tumor aggressiveness. PD-L1 expression in HCC has recently been characterized and its crucial role in HCC progression has been strongly suggested [14].

Interestingly, it has been observed in HCC patient cohort that even with increased peripheral and intratumor PD-1 expression on $CD8^+$ T cells, tumor cells were also rich in PD-L1 expression. These findings thus showed a correlation between a high PD-L1 expression within the tumor and a poorer outcome with early HCC recurrence after liver resection because of the induction of $CD8^+$ T cell apoptosis [120]. The challenges of next studies will be to determine the mechanisms by which tumors promote PD-L1 expression on tumor cells and to find strategies to bypass the inhibitory signal delivered to PD-1 expressing cells including CD8+ T lymphocytes.

9.3.2.2 IL-17-producing Cells

IL-17 is in majority produced by Th17 lymphocytes and targets a large variety of cells through its ubiquitously expressed receptor IL-17RA. However, other IL-17-producing cell types have been identified including $\gamma\delta$ T cells or neutrophils [113]. It has been reported that in HCC IL-17 levels were increased compared to non-tumor tissues [89]. Furthermore, a positive correlation has been established between high expression of IL-17 and microvessel density in tissues and poor survival in patients with HCC [143] suggesting that IL-17 may promote HCC growth by promoting angiogenesis.

In addition, neutrophils detected inside HCC tumors are associated with a poor recurrence-free survival for patients with HCC after liver resection. Peritumoral neutrophils promote angiogenesis leading therefore to stimulate tumor growth [81, 82]. More surprisingly, a study has shown that IL-17 can recruit neutrophils. Peritumoral tissue was also found enriched in Th17 lymphocytes which number is correlated with tumor activated monocytes that have been reported to induce IL-17 producing cells proliferation [81, 82]. Despite the positive correlation between IL-17 producing cells and poor survival in HCC patients, the underlying mechanisms by which these cells lead to HCC progression remain poorly defined.

9.3.2.3 Inflammation-Induced Epithelial Mesenchymal Transition (EMT)

Physiologically, EMT is a key step during embryogenesis, pathological events, inflammation but it can also trigger metastasis development in cancer context [9, 70]. During this process, morphological modifications occurs in epithelial cells which adopt a fibroblast-like phenotype. Through a complex cytoskeleton reorganization, many intercellular junctions characterizing epithelial cells are lost such as desmosomes, adherent junctions, tight junctions and gap junctions. EMT thus promotes epithelial markers loss including E-cadherin in favor of an induction of fibroblast markers such as fibronectin, matrix metalloproteinase. Such transformation allows those transformed cells to leave the original tissue and colonize other tissue through the blood circulation. TGF-β is one of the most relevant inflammatory mediator involved in EMT. It is considered as a key factor in embryogenesis but also in fibrosis and cancer development in many models [35, 138] through SMAD2, SMAD3 and SMAD4 [119, 129]. Studies have brought evidence that inflammation promotes EMT via the induction of pro-inflammatory cytokines. It has been shown that together TNF-α and IL-6 enhance TGF-β signaling pathways which stimulate EMT [7]. These two cytokines are known to trigger NF-κB which induces many factors implicated in EMT. Lastly, ROS synthesis has also been shown to induce EMT [131]. Exploring more deeply the involvement of cytokines in EMT in a context of CHC could open new therapeutic options.

9.4 HCC Therapeutic Failure and Cytokine-Based Therapy

At late stage, patients are not eligible for surgical resection of the tumor or for liver transplant, and the efficacy of classical radiotherapy and chimiotherapy is very poor. Since 2008, the SHARP (Sorafenib HCC Assessment Randomised Protocol) trials combining multikinase inhibitory and anti-angiogenic properties is considered as a standard for advanced HCC and showed an improved overall survival in Child–Pugh class A patients with advanced HCC upon treatment. HCC-patients given Sorafenib have a longer progression-free survival (PFS) with a median overall survival reaching 10.7 months in sorafenib treated patients vs 7.9 months in the placebo patients [90] Moreover, the high capacity of resistance of CSC to sorafenib therapy suggests that CSCs may contribute to the poor prognosis.

In HCC many cytokine levels are deregulated leading to promote or inhibit carcinogenesis. The development of combined therapy like IFN-α with ribavirin has markedly reduced HCC incidence. However antiviral therapies only help to delay the development of HCC. More and more anti-tumor therapeutic options use strategies to regulate cytokines levels or modulate immune cell activity. Loco-regional immune-chemotherapy based on lymphokine-activated killer cells (LAK) is a relevant approach in HCC treatment. LAKs release many cytokines including IFN-γ, IL-2 and IL-12 promoting cytolytic activity against tumor cells [78]. Many studies also proposed to enhance cytokine responses and more specifically to the liver. A murine HCC model was developed with adenoviral vector carrying IL-12 leading to reduce tumor growth and induce immune infiltration potentially responsible for the inhibition of angiogenesis [2]. Consistently, IL-12 intrahepatic administration in BALB/c has shown early infiltration of lymphocytes and macrophages resulting in a reduction of tumor progression [108]. Furthermore, combined immunotherapy in a murine model of HCC based on IL-12 and GM-CSF triggered a powerful antitumor response and avoid the side-effect of IL-12 treatment alone [132].

9.5 Conclusion

Although liver inflammation is critical for protection against infections and for triggering liver regeneration mechanisms, it must be finely tuned and "turned off" right after the clearance of the pathogens and the achievement of tissue repair. Indeed, excessive and recurrent liver inflammation is a common process observed in livers of alcoholic patients and in non-alcoholic steatohepatitis, in drug and chemical intoxication, during viral and bacterial infection, as well as in certain idiopathic liver pathologies such as autoimmune hepatitis. A high variety of immune cells can infiltrate the liver tissue (Fig. 9.2). Their quantity and their activity defined by their ability to produce a large spectrum of cytokines, depend on the underlying chronic liver disease. One of the major challenges in the liver field is to understand the cellular and molecular mechanisms underlying the chronic inflammatory processes associated with acute and chronic injury. The recent advances in immunology field

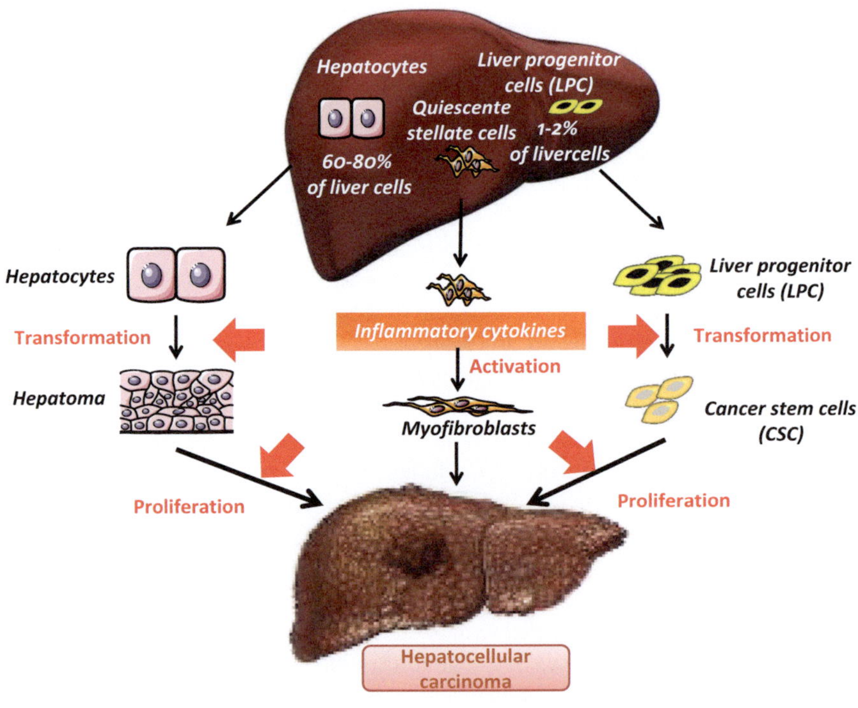

Fig. 9.2 Influence of cytokines in HCC initiation and progression. Inflammatory cytokines are responsible for stellate cell activation and fibrosis development (IL-6, TGF-b, IL-1b), liver progenitor cell expansion (IL-6, TNF-a, IL-22) and DNA alteration via ROS production

sheds some light on the important role of cytokine milieu in which tumoral cells can emerge and proliferate. This also demonstrates how complex and heterogeneous is the liver inflammatory response according to the etiology leading to HCC. This strongly suggests that a better characterization of the inflammatory process would allow developing a personalized medicine for patients, and would constitute a promising strategy in HCC prevention and cure.

References

1. Akriviadis E, Botla R, Briggs W, Han S, Reynolds T, Shakil O. Pentoxifylline improves short-term survival in severe acute alcoholic hepatitis: a double-blind, placebo-controlled trial. Gastroenterology. 2000;119(6):1637–48.
2. Andrews KJ, Ribas A, Butterfield LH, Vollmer CM, Eilber FC, Dissette VB, Nelson SD, Shintaku P, Mekhoubad S, Nakayama T, Taniguchi M, Glaspy JA, McBride WH, Economou JS. Adenovirus-interleukin-12-mediated tumor regression in a murine hepatocellular carcinoma model is not dependent on CD1-restricted natural killer T cells. Cancer Res. 2000;60(22):6457–64.
3. Aoudjehane L, Pissaia A Jr, Scatton O, Podevin P, Massault PP, Chouzenoux S, Soubrane O, Calmus Y, Conti F. Interleukin-4 induces the activation and collagen production of cultured human intrahepatic fibroblasts via the STAT-6 pathway. Lab Investig. 2008;88(9):973–85.
4. Avila MA, Berasain C, Sangro B, Prieto J. New therapies for hepatocellular carcinoma. Oncogene. 2006;25(27):3866–84.
5. Bai S, Nasser MW, Wang B, Hsu SH, Datta J, Kutay H, Yadav A, Nuovo G, Kumar P, Ghoshal K. MicroRNA-122 inhibits tumorigenic properties of hepatocellular carcinoma cells and sensitizes these cells to sorafenib. J Biol Chem. 2009;284(46):32015–27.
6. Baik M, Yu JH, Hennighausen L. Growth hormone-STAT5 regulation of growth, hepatocellular carcinoma, and liver metabolism. Ann N Y Acad Sci. 2011;1229:29–37.
7. Bates RC, Mercurio AM. Tumor necrosis factor-alpha stimulates the epithelial-to-mesenchymal transition of human colonic organoids. Mol Biol Cell. 2003;14(5):1790–800.
8. Batey RG, Wang J. Molecular pathogenesis of T lymphocyte-induced liver injury in alcoholic hepatitis. Front Biosci. 2002;7:d1662–75.
9. Baum B, Settleman J, Quinlan MP. Transitions between epithelial and mesenchymal states in development and disease. Semin Cell Dev Biol. 2008;19(3):294–308.
10. Beckebaum S, Zhang X, Chen X, Yu Z, Frilling A, Dworacki G, Grosse-Wilde H, Broelsch CE, Gerken G, Cicinnati VR. Increased levels of interleukin-10 in serum from patients with hepatocellular carcinoma correlate with profound numerical deficiencies and immature phenotype of circulating dendritic cell subsets. Clin Cancer Res. 2004;10(21):7260–9.
11. Benoit M, Barbarat B, Bernard A, Olive D, Mege JL. Coxiella burnetii, the agent of Q fever, stimulates an atypical M2 activation program in human macrophages. Eur J Immunol. 2008;38(4):1065–70.
12. Bode C, Bode JC. Activation of the innate immune system and alcoholic liver disease: effects of ethanol per se or enhanced intestinal translocation of bacterial toxins induced by ethanol? Alcohol Clin Exp Res. 2005;29(11 Suppl):166S–71S.
13. Boetticher NC, Peine CJ, Kwo P, Abrams GA, Patel T, Aqel B, Boardman L, Gores GJ, Harmsen WS, McClain CJ, Kamath PS, Shah VH. A randomized, double-blinded, placebo-controlled multicenter trial of etanercept in the treatment of alcoholic hepatitis. Gastroenterology. 2008;135(6):1953–60.
14. Calderaro J, Rousseau B, Amaddeo G, Mercey M, Charpy C, Costentin C, Luciani A, Zafrani ES, Laurent A, Azoulay D, Lafdil F, Pawlotsky JM. Programmed death ligand 1 expression

in hepatocellular carcinoma: relationship with clinical and pathological features. Hepatology. 2016;64(6):2038–46.
15. Calin GA, Croce CM. MicroRNA signatures in human cancers. Nat Rev Cancer. 2006;6(11):857–66.
16. Callegari E, Elamin BK, Giannone F, Milazzo M, Altavilla G, Fornari F, Giacomelli L, D'Abundo L, Ferracin M, Bassi C, Zagatti B, Corra F, Miotto E, Lupini L, Bolondi L, Gramantieri L, Croce CM, Sabbioni S, Negrini M. Liver tumorigenicity promoted by microRNA-221 in a mouse transgenic model. Hepatology. 2012;56(3):1025–33.
17. Cao Q, Batey R, Pang G, Clancy R. Altered T-lymphocyte responsiveness to polyclonal cell activators is responsible for liver cell necrosis in alcohol-fed rats. Alcohol Clin Exp Res. 1998;22(3):723–9.
18. Chang HD, Radbruch A. The pro- and anti-inflammatory potential of interleukin-12. Ann N Y Acad Sci. 2007;1109:40–6.
19. Chen J, Katz LH, Munoz NM, Gu S, Shin JH, Jogunoori WS, Lee MH, Belkin MD, Kim SB, White JC, Andricovich J, Tzatsos A, Li S, Kim SS, Shetty K, Mishra B, Rashid A, Lee JS, Mishra L. Vitamin D deficiency promotes liver tumor growth in transforming growth factor-beta/Smad3-deficient mice through Wnt and toll-like receptor 7 pathway modulation. Sci Rep. 2016;6:30217.
20. Chen RH, Su YH, Chuang RL, Chang TY. Suppression of transforming growth factor-beta-induced apoptosis through a phosphatidylinositol 3-kinase/Akt-dependent pathway. Oncogene. 1998;17(15):1959–68.
21. Chia CS, Ban K, Ithnin H, Singh H, Krishnan R, Mokhtar S, Malihan N, Seow HF. Expression of interleukin-18, interferon-gamma and interleukin-10 in hepatocellular carcinoma. Immunol Lett. 2002;84(3):163–72.
22. Colnot S, Decaens T, Niwa-Kawakita M, Godard C, Hamard G, Kahn A, Giovannini M, Perret C. Liver-targeted disruption of Apc in mice activates beta-catenin signaling and leads to hepatocellular carcinomas. Proc Natl Acad Sci U S A. 2004a;101(49):17216–21.
23. Colnot S, Niwa-Kawakita M, Hamard G, Godard C, Le Plenier S, Houbron C, Romagnolo B, Berrebi D, Giovannini M, Perret C. Colorectal cancers in a new mouse model of familial adenomatous polyposis: influence of genetic and environmental modifiers. Lab Investig. 2004b;84(12):1619–30.
24. Corzo CA, Condamine T, Lu L, Cotter MJ, Youn JI, Cheng P, Cho HI, Celis E, Quiceno DG, Padhya T, McCaffrey TV, McCaffrey JC, Gabrilovich DI. HIF-1alpha regulates function and differentiation of myeloid-derived suppressor cells in the tumor microenvironment. J Exp Med. 2010;207(11):2439–53.
25. Coulouarn C, Factor VM, Andersen JB, Durkin ME, Thorgeirsson SS. Loss of miR-122 expression in liver cancer correlates with suppression of the hepatic phenotype and gain of metastatic properties. Oncogene. 2009;28(40):3526–36.
26. Cui Y, Hosui A, Sun R, Shen K, Gavrilova O, Chen W, Cam MC, Gao B, Robinson GW, Hennighausen L. Loss of signal transducer and activator of transcription 5 leads to hepatosteatosis and impaired liver regeneration. Hepatology. 2007;46(2):504–13.
27. Curtis BJ, Zahs A, Kovacs EJ. Epigenetic targets for reversing immune defects caused by alcohol exposure. Alcohol Res. 2013;35(1):97–113.
28. Cussigh A, Falleti E, Fabris C, Bitetto D, Cmet S, Fontanini E, Bignulin S, Fornasiere E, Fumolo E, Minisini R, Pirisi M, Toniutto P. Interleukin 6 promoter polymorphisms influence the outcome of chronic hepatitis C. Immunogenetics. 2011;63(1):33–41.
29. Davies RA, Knight B, Tian YW, Yeoh GC, Olynyk JK. Hepatic oval cell response to the choline-deficient, ethionine supplemented model of murine liver injury is attenuated by the administration of a cyclo-oxygenase 2 inhibitor. Carcinogenesis. 2006;27(8):1607–16.
30. de La Coste A, Romagnolo B, Billuart P, Renard CA, Buendia MA, Soubrane O, Fabre M, Chelly J, Beldjord C, Kahn A, Perret C. Somatic mutations of the beta-catenin gene are frequent in mouse and human hepatocellular carcinomas. Proc Natl Acad Sci U S A. 1998;95(15):8847–51.

31. De Larco JE, Wuertz BR, Furcht LT. The potential role of neutrophils in promoting the metastatic phenotype of tumors releasing interleukin-8. Clin Cancer Res. 2004;10(15):4895–900.
32. Dogru T, Ercin CN, Erdem G, Sonmez A, Tapan S, Tasci I. Increased hepatic and circulating interleukin-6 levels in human nonalcoholic steatohepatitis. Am J Gastroenterol. 2008;103(12):3217–8.
33. Dondeti MF, El-Maadawy EA, Talaat RM. Hepatitis-related hepatocellular carcinoma: insights into cytokine gene polymorphisms. World J Gastroenterol. 2016;22(30):6800–16.
34. El-Omar EM, Carrington M, Chow WH, McColl KE, Bream JH, Young HA, Herrera J, Lissowska J, Yuan CC, Rothman N, Lanyon G, Martin M, Fraumeni JF Jr, Rabkin CS. Interleukin-1 polymorphisms associated with increased risk of gastric cancer. Nature. 2000;404(6776):398–402.
35. Ellenrieder V, Fernandez Zapico ME, Urrutia R. TGFbeta-mediated signaling and transcriptional regulation in pancreatic development and cancer. Curr Opin Gastroenterol. 2001;17(5):434–40.
36. Espanol-Suner R, Carpentier R, Van Hul N, Legry V, Achouri Y, Cordi S, Jacquemin P, Lemaigre F, Leclercq IA. Liver progenitor cells yield functional hepatocytes in response to chronic liver injury in mice. Gastroenterology. 2012;143(6):1564–75. e1567
37. Farah IO, Mola PW, Kariuki TM, Nyindo M, Blanton RE, King CL. Repeated exposure induces periportal fibrosis in Schistosoma Mansoni-infected baboons: role of TGF-beta and IL-4. J Immunol. 2000;164(10):5337–43.
38. Fiorentino DF, Bond MW, Mosmann TR. Two types of mouse T helper cell. IV. Th2 clones secrete a factor that inhibits cytokine production by Th1 clones. J Exp Med. 1989;170(6):2081–95.
39. Flecken T, Schmidt N, Hild S, Gostick E, Drognitz O, Zeiser R, Schemmer P, Bruns H, Eiermann T, Price DA, Blum HE, Neumann-Haefelin C, Thimme R. Immunodominance and functional alterations of tumor-associated antigen-specific CD8+ T-cell responses in hepatocellular carcinoma. Hepatology. 2014;59(4):1415–26.
40. Fornari F, Gramantieri L, Giovannini C, Veronese A, Ferracin M, Sabbioni S, Calin GA, Grazi GL, Croce CM, Tavolari S, Chieco P, Negrini M, Bolondi L. MiR-122/cyclin G1 interaction modulates p53 activity and affects doxorubicin sensitivity of human hepatocarcinoma cells. Cancer Res. 2009;69(14):5761–7.
41. Forner A, Bruix J. Biomarkers for early diagnosis of hepatocellular carcinoma. Lancet Oncol. 2012;13(8):750–1.
42. Freeman GJ, Long AJ, Iwai Y, Bourque K, Chernova T, Nishimura H, Fitz LJ, Malenkovich N, Okazaki T, Byrne MC, Horton HF, Fouser L, Carter L, Ling V, Bowman MR, Carreno BM, Collins M, Wood CR, Honjo T. Engagement of the PD-1 immunoinhibitory receptor by a novel B7 family member leads to negative regulation of lymphocyte activation. J Exp Med. 2000;192(7):1027–34.
43. Friedbichler K, Themanns M, Mueller KM, Schlederer M, Kornfeld JW, Terracciano LM, Kozlov AV, Haindl S, Kenner L, Kolbe T, Mueller M, Snibson KJ, Heim MH, Moriggl R. Growth-hormone-induced signal transducer and activator of transcription 5 signaling causes gigantism, inflammation, and premature death but protects mice from aggressive liver cancer. Hepatology. 2012;55(3):941–52.
44. Gabrilovich D. Mechanisms and functional significance of tumour-induced dendritic-cell defects. Nat Rev Immunol. 2004;4(12):941–52.
45. Galdiero MR, Bonavita E, Barajon I, Garlanda C, Mantovani A, Jaillon S. Tumor associated macrophages and neutrophils in cancer. Immunobiology. 2013;218(11):1402–10.
46. Gao Q, Qiu SJ, Fan J, Zhou J, Wang XY, Xiao YS, Xu Y, Li YW, Tang ZY. Intratumoral balance of regulatory and cytotoxic T cells is associated with prognosis of hepatocellular carcinoma after resection. J Clin Oncol. 2007;25(18):2586–93.
47. Garofalo M, Di Leva G, Romano G, Nuovo G, Suh SS, Ngankeu A, Taccioli C, Pichiorri F, Alder H, Secchiero P, Gasparini P, Gonelli A, Costinean S, Acunzo M, Condorelli G, Croce CM. miR-221&222 regulate TRAIL resistance and enhance tumorigenicity through PTEN and TIMP3 downregulation. Cancer Cell. 2009;16(6):498–509.

48. Gedaly R, Angulo P, Hundley J, Daily MF, Chen C, Koch A, Evers BM. PI-103 and sorafenib inhibit hepatocellular carcinoma cell proliferation by blocking Ras/Raf/MAPK and PI3K/AKT/mTOR pathways. Anticancer Res. 2010;30(12):4951–8.
49. Gehring AJ, Ho ZZ, Tan AT, Aung MO, Lee KH, Tan KC, Lim SG, Bertoletti A. Profile of tumor antigen-specific CD8 T cells in patients with hepatitis B virus-related hepatocellular carcinoma. Gastroenterology. 2009;137(2):682–90.
50. Giannelli G, Fransvea E, Marinosci F, Bergamini C, Colucci S, Schiraldi O, Antonaci S. Transforming growth factor-beta1 triggers hepatocellular carcinoma invasiveness via alpha3beta1 integrin. Am J Pathol. 2002;161(1):183–93.
51. Gramantieri L, Ferracin M, Fornari F, Veronese A, Sabbioni S, Liu CG, Calin GA, Giovannini C, Ferrazzi E, Grazi GL, Croce CM, Bolondi L, Negrini M. Cyclin G1 is a target of miR-122a, a microRNA frequently down-regulated in human hepatocellular carcinoma. Cancer Res. 2007;67(13):6092–9.
52. Guillot A, Hamdaoui N, Bizy A, Zoltani K, Souktani R, Zafrani ES, Mallat A, Lotersztajn S, Lafdil F. Cannabinoid receptor 2 counteracts interleukin-17-induced immune and fibrogenic responses in mouse liver. Hepatology. 2014;59(1):296–306.
53. Gungor N, Knaapen AM, Munnia A, Peluso M, Haenen GR, Chiu RK, Godschalk RW, van Schooten FJ. Genotoxic effects of neutrophils and hypochlorous acid. Mutagenesis. 2010;25(2):149–54.
54. Hagiwara S, Kudo M, Nagai T, Inoue T, Ueshima K, Nishida N, Watanabe T, Sakurai T. Activation of JNK and high expression level of CD133 predict a poor response to sorafenib in hepatocellular carcinoma. Br J Cancer. 2012;106(12):1997–2003.
55. Hanahan D, Weinberg RA. Hallmarks of cancer: the next generation. Cell. 2011;144(5):646–74.
56. Harada N, Oshima H, Katoh M, Tamai Y, Oshima M, Taketo MM. Hepatocarcinogenesis in mice with beta-catenin and Ha-ras gene mutations. Cancer Res. 2004a;64(1):48–54.
57. Harada N, Shimada M, Okano S, Suehiro T, Soejima Y, Tomita Y, Maehara Y. IL-12 gene therapy is an effective therapeutic strategy for hepatocellular carcinoma in immunosuppressed mice. J Immunol. 2004b;173(11):6635–44.
58. Hirano S, Iwashita Y, Sasaki A, Kai S, Ohta M, Kitano S. Increased mRNA expression of chemokines in hepatocellular carcinoma with tumor-infiltrating lymphocytes. J Gastroenterol Hepatol. 2007;22(5):690–6.
59. Hiroishi K, Eguchi J, Baba T, Shimazaki T, Ishii S, Hiraide A, Sakaki M, Doi H, Uozumi S, Omori R, Matsumura T, Yanagawa T, Ito T, Imawari M. Strong CD8(+) T-cell responses against tumor-associated antigens prolong the recurrence-free interval after tumor treatment in patients with hepatocellular carcinoma. J Gastroenterol. 2010;45(4):451–8.
60. Horiguchi N, Ishac EJ, Gao B. Liver regeneration is suppressed in alcoholic cirrhosis: correlation with decreased STAT3 activation. Alcohol. 2007;41(4):271–80.
61. Horiike S, Kawanishi S, Kaito M, Ma N, Tanaka H, Fujita N, Iwasa M, Kobayashi Y, Hiraku Y, Oikawa S, Murata M, Wang J, Semba R, Watanabe S, Adachi Y. Accumulation of 8-nitroguanine in the liver of patients with chronic hepatitis C. J Hepatol. 2005;43(3):403–10.
62. Hosui A, Kimura A, Yamaji D, Zhu BM, Na R, Hennighausen L. Loss of STAT5 causes liver fibrosis and cancer development through increased TGF-{beta} and STAT3 activation. J Exp Med. 2009;206(4):819–31.
63. Hou J, Lin L, Zhou W, Wang Z, Ding G, Dong Q, Qin L, Wu X, Zheng Y, Yang Y, Tian W, Zhang Q, Wang C, Zhang Q, Zhuang SM, Zheng L, Liang A, Tao W, Cao X. Identification of miRNomes in human liver and hepatocellular carcinoma reveals miR-199a/b-3p as therapeutic target for hepatocellular carcinoma. Cancer Cell. 2011;19(2):232–43.
64. Hsu SH, Wang B, Kota J, Yu J, Costinean S, Kutay H, Yu L, Bai S, La Perle K, Chivukula RR, Mao H, Wei M, Clark KR, Mendell JR, Caligiuri MA, Jacob ST, Mendell JT, Ghoshal K. Essential metabolic, anti-inflammatory, and anti-tumorigenic functions of miR-122 in liver. J Clin Invest. 2012;122(8):2871–83.
65. Hussain SP, Schwank J, Staib F, Wang XW, Harris CC. TP53 mutations and hepatocellular carcinoma: insights into the etiology and pathogenesis of liver cancer. Oncogene. 2007;26(15):2166–76.

66. Inagaki Y, Nemoto T, Kushida M, Sheng Y, Higashi K, Ikeda K, Kawada N, Shirasaki F, Takehara K, Sugiyama K, Fujii M, Yamauchi H, Nakao A, de Crombrugghe B, Watanabe T, Okazaki I. Interferon alfa down-regulates collagen gene transcription and suppresses experimental hepatic fibrosis in mice. Hepatology. 2003;38(4):890–9.
67. Jeong WI, Park O, Radaeva S, Gao B. STAT1 inhibits liver fibrosis in mice by inhibiting stellate cell proliferation and stimulating NK cell cytotoxicity. Hepatology. 2006;44(6):1441–51.
68. Jia XQ, Cheng HQ, Qian X, Bian CX, Shi ZM, Zhang JP, Jiang BH, Feng ZQ. Lentivirus-mediated overexpression of microRNA-199a inhibits cell proliferation of human hepatocellular carcinoma. Cell Biochem Biophys. 2012;62(1):237–44.
69. Jin Z, Sun R, Wei H, Gao X, Chen Y, Tian Z. Accelerated liver fibrosis in hepatitis B virus transgenic mice: involvement of natural killer T cells. Hepatology. 2011;53(1):219–29.
70. Kalluri R, Weinberg RA. The basics of epithelial-mesenchymal transition. J Clin Invest. 2009;119(6):1420–8.
71. Kaplan MH, Whitfield JR, Boros DL, Grusby MJ. Th2 cells are required for the Schistosoma Mansoni egg-induced granulomatous response. J Immunol. 1998;160(4):1850–6.
72. Karin M, Lawrence T, Nizet V. Innate immunity gone awry: linking microbial infections to chronic inflammation and cancer. Cell. 2006;124(4):823–35.
73. Knight B, Tirnitz-Parker JE, Olynyk JK. C-kit inhibition by imatinib mesylate attenuates progenitor cell expansion and inhibits liver tumor formation in mice. Gastroenterology. 2008;135(3):969–79. 979 e961
74. Kobayashi N, Hiraoka N, Yamagami W, Ojima H, Kanai Y, Kosuge T, Nakajima A, Hirohashi S. FOXP3+ regulatory T cells affect the development and progression of hepatocarcinogenesis. Clin Cancer Res. 2007;13(3):902–11.
75. Kolch W. Meaningful relationships: the regulation of the Ras/Raf/MEK/ERK pathway by protein interactions. Biochem J. 2000;351(Pt 2):289–305.
76. Komita H, Homma S, Saotome H, Zeniya M, Ohno T, Toda G. Interferon-gamma produced by interleukin-12-activated tumor infiltrating CD8+T cells directly induces apoptosis of mouse hepatocellular carcinoma. J Hepatol. 2006;45(5):662–72.
77. Kono H, Uesugi T, Froh M, Rusyn I, Bradford BU, Thurman RG. ICAM-1 is involved in the mechanism of alcohol-induced liver injury: studies with knockout mice. Am J Physiol Gastrointest Liver Physiol. 2001;280(6):G1289–95.
78. Kountouras J, Boura P, Kouklakis G. Locoregional immunochemotherapy in hepatocellular carcinoma. Hepato-Gastroenterology. 2002;49(46):1109–12.
79. Kovalovich K, DeAngelis RA, Li W, Furth EE, Ciliberto G, Taub R. Increased toxin-induced liver injury and fibrosis in interleukin-6-deficient mice. Hepatology. 2000;31(1):149–59.
80. Kroy DC, Beraza N, Tschaharganeh DF, Sander LE, Erschfeld S, Giebeler A, Liedtke C, Wasmuth HE, Trautwein C, Streetz KL. Lack of interleukin-6/glycoprotein 130/signal transducers and activators of transcription-3 signaling in hepatocytes predisposes to liver steatosis and injury in mice. Hepatology. 2010;51(2):463–73.
81. Kuang DM, Peng C, Zhao Q, Wu Y, Chen MS, Zheng L. Activated monocytes in peritumoral stroma of hepatocellular carcinoma promote expansion of memory T helper 17 cells. Hepatology. 2010a;51(1):154–64.
82. Kuang DM, Peng C, Zhao Q, Wu Y, Zhu LY, Wang J, Yin XY, Li L, Zheng L. Tumor-activated monocytes promote expansion of IL-17-producing CD8+ T cells in hepatocellular carcinoma patients. J Immunol. 2010b;185(3):1544–9.
83. Kuang DM, Zhao Q, Wu Y, Peng C, Wang J, Xu Z, Yin XY, Zheng L. Peritumoral neutrophils link inflammatory response to disease progression by fostering angiogenesis in hepatocellular carcinoma. J Hepatol. 2011;54(5):948–55.
84. Lafdil F, Miller AM, Ki SH, Gao B. Th17 cells and their associated cytokines in liver diseases. Cell Mol Immunol. 2010;7(4):250–4.
85. Lee HC, Tian B, Sedivy JM, Wands JR, Kim M. Loss of Raf kinase inhibitor protein promotes cell proliferation and migration of human hepatoma cells. Gastroenterology. 2006;131(4):1208–17.

86. Lee TK, Cheung VC, Ng IO. Liver tumor-initiating cells as a therapeutic target for hepatocellular carcinoma. Cancer Lett. 2012;338(1):101–9.
87. Lee TK, Cheung VC, Ng IO. Liver tumor-initiating cells as a therapeutic target for hepatocellular carcinoma. Cancer Lett. 2013;338(1):101–9.
88. Lemmers A, Moreno C, Gustot T, Marechal R, Degre D, Demetter P, de Nadai P, Geerts A, Quertinmont E, Vercruysse V, Le Moine O, Deviere J. The interleukin-17 pathway is involved in human alcoholic liver disease. Hepatology. 2009;49(2):646–57.
89. Liao R, Sun J, Wu H, Yi Y, Wang JX, He HW, Cai XY, Zhou J, Cheng YF, Fan J, Qiu SJ. High expression of IL-17 and IL-17RE associate with poor prognosis of hepatocellular carcinoma. J Exp Clin Cancer Res. 2013;32:3.
90. Llovet JM, Ricci S, Mazzaferro V, Hilgard P, Gane E, Blanc JF, de Oliveira AC, Santoro A, Raoul JL, Forner A, Schwartz M, Porta C, Zeuzem S, Bolondi L, Greten TF, Galle PR, Seitz JF, Borbath I, Haussinger D, Giannaris T, Shan M, Moscovici M, Voliotis D, Bruix J, S. I. S. Group. Sorafenib in advanced hepatocellular carcinoma. N Engl J Med. 2008;359(4):378–90.
91. Luedde T, Schwabe RF. NF-kappaB in the liver–linking injury, fibrosis and hepatocellular carcinoma. Nat Rev Gastroenterol Hepatol. 2011;8(2):108–18.
92. Maeda S, Kamata H, Luo JL, Leffert H, Karin M. IKKbeta couples hepatocyte death to cytokine-driven compensatory proliferation that promotes chemical hepatocarcinogenesis. Cell. 2005;121(7):977–90.
93. Mantovani A. The yin-yang of tumor-associated neutrophils. Cancer Cell. 2009;16(3):173–4.
94. Marquardt JU, Raggi C, Andersen JB, Seo D, Avital I, Geller D, Lee YH, Kitade M, Holczbauer A, Gillen MC, Conner EA, Factor VM, Thorgeirsson SS. Human hepatic cancer stem cells are characterized by common stemness traits and diverse oncogenic pathways. Hepatology. 2011;54(3):1031–42.
95. McClain CJ, Song Z, Barve SS, Hill DB, Deaciuc I. Recent advances in alcoholic liver disease. IV. Dysregulated cytokine metabolism in alcoholic liver disease. Am J Physiol Gastrointest Liver Physiol. 2004;287(3):G497–502.
96. Medina R, Zaidi SK, Liu CG, Stein JL, van Wijnen AJ, Croce CM, Stein GS. MicroRNAs 221 and 222 bypass quiescence and compromise cell survival. Cancer Res. 2008;68(8):2773–80.
97. Mentink-Kane MM, Cheever AW, Wilson MS, Madala SK, Beers LM, Ramalingam TR, Wynn TA. Accelerated and progressive and lethal liver fibrosis in mice that lack interleukin (IL)-10, IL-12p40, and IL-13Ralpha2. Gastroenterology. 2011;141(6):2200–9.
98. Mishra L, Banker T, Murray J, Byers S, Thenappan A, He AR, Shetty K, Johnson L, Reddy EP. Liver stem cells and hepatocellular carcinoma. Hepatology. 2009;49(1):318–29.
99. Mosmann TR, Coffman RL. TH1 and TH2 cells: different patterns of lymphokine secretion lead to different functional properties. Annu Rev Immunol. 1989;7:145–73.
100. Mueller KM, Kornfeld JW, Friedbichler K, Blaas L, Egger G, Esterbauer H, Hasselblatt P, Schlederer M, Haindl S, Wagner KU, Engblom D, Haemmerle G, Kratky D, Sexl V, Kenner L, Kozlov AV, Terracciano L, Zechner R, Schuetz G, Casanova E, Pospisilik JA, Heim MH, Moriggl R. Impairment of hepatic growth hormone and glucocorticoid receptor signaling causes steatosis and hepatocellular carcinoma in mice. Hepatology. 2011;54(4):1398–409.
101. Murata M, Thanan R, Ma N, Kawanishi S. Role of nitrative and oxidative DNA damage in inflammation-related carcinogenesis. J Biomed Biotechnol. 2012;2012:623019.
102. Nagy LE. The role of innate immunity in alcoholic liver disease. Alcohol Res. 2015;37(2):237–50.
103. Narita Y, Wakita D, Ohkur T, Chamoto K, Nishimura T. Potential differentiation of tumor bearing mouse CD11b+gr-1+ immature myeloid cells into both suppressor macrophages and immunostimulatory dendritic cells. Biomed Res. 2009;30(1):7–15.
104. Naveau S, Chollet-Martin S, Dharancy S, Mathurin P, Jouet P, Piquet MA, Davion T, Oberti F, Broet P, Emilie D, F. Foie-Alcool group of the Association Francaise pour l'Etude du. A double-blind randomized controlled trial of infliximab associated with prednisolone in acute alcoholic hepatitis. Hepatology. 2004;39(5):1390–7.

105. Negrini M, Gramantieri L, Sabbioni S, Croce CM. microRNA involvement in hepatocellular carcinoma. Anti Cancer Agents Med Chem. 2011;11(6):500–21.
106. Park EJ, Lee JH, Yu GY, He G, Ali SR, Holzer RG, Osterreicher CH, Takahashi H, Karin M. Dietary and genetic obesity promote liver inflammation and tumorigenesis by enhancing IL-6 and TNF expression. Cell. 2010;140(2):197–208.
107. Paul WE, Seder RA. Lymphocyte responses and cytokines. Cell. 1994;76(2):241–51.
108. Peron JM, Couderc B, Rochaix P, Douin-Echinard V, Asnacios A, Souque A, Voigt JJ, Buscail L, Vinel JP, Favre G. Treatment of murine hepatocellular carcinoma using genetically modified cells to express interleukin-12. J Gastroenterol Hepatol. 2004;19(4):388–96.
109. Plum W, Tschaharganeh DF, Kroy DC, Corsten E, Erschfeld S, Dierssen U, Wasmuth H, Trautwein C, Streetz KL. Lack of glycoprotein 130/signal transducer and activator of transcription 3-mediated signaling in hepatocytes enhances chronic liver injury and fibrosis progression in a model of sclerosing cholangitis. Am J Pathol. 2010;176(5):2236–46.
110. Polakis P. The oncogenic activation of beta-catenin. Curr Opin Genet Dev. 1999;9(1):15–21.
111. Rachmilewitz D, Stamler JS, Bachwich D, Karmeli F, Ackerman Z, Podolsky DK. Enhanced colonic nitric oxide generation and nitric oxide synthase activity in ulcerative colitis and Crohn's disease. Gut. 1995;36(5):718–23.
112. Radaeva S, Sun R, Jaruga B, Nguyen VT, Tian Z, Gao B. Natural killer cells ameliorate liver fibrosis by killing activated stellate cells in NKG2D-dependent and tumor necrosis factor-related apoptosis-inducing ligand-dependent manners. Gastroenterology. 2006;130(2):435–52.
113. Rajoriya N, Fergusson JR, Leithead JA, Klenerman P. Gamma Delta T-lymphocytes in hepatitis C and chronic liver disease. Front Immunol. 2014;5:400.
114. Ramadori G, Christ B. Cytokines and the hepatic acute-phase response. Semin Liver Dis. 1999;19(2):141–55.
115. Rambaldi A, Gluud C. S-adenosyl-L-methionine for alcoholic liver diseases. Cochrane Database Syst Rev. 2006;2:CD002235.
116. Rieder G, Hofmann JA, Hatz RA, Stolte M, Enders GA. Up-regulation of inducible nitric oxide synthase in helicobacter pylori-associated gastritis may represent an increased risk factor to develop gastric carcinoma of the intestinal type. Int J Med Microbiol. 2003;293(6):403–12.
117. Rountree CB, Mishra L, Willenbring H. Stem cells in liver diseases and cancer: recent advances on the path to new therapies. Hepatology. 2012;55(1):298–306.
118. Sakaguchi S. Naturally arising CD4+ regulatory t cells for immunologic self-tolerance and negative control of immune responses. Annu Rev Immunol. 2004;22:531–62.
119. Sato M, Muragaki Y, Saika S, Roberts AB, Ooshima A. Targeted disruption of TGF-beta1/Smad3 signaling protects against renal tubulointerstitial fibrosis induced by unilateral ureteral obstruction. J Clin Invest. 2003;112(10):1486–94.
120. Shi F, Shi M, Zeng Z, Qi RZ, Liu ZW, Zhang JY, Yang YP, Tien P, Wang FS. PD-1 and PD-L1 upregulation promotes CD8(+) T-cell apoptosis and postoperative recurrence in hepatocellular carcinoma patients. Int J Cancer. 2011;128(4):887–96.
121. Sozio M, Crabb DW. Alcohol and lipid metabolism. Am J Physiol Endocrinol Metab. 2008;295(1):E10–6.
122. Sripa B, Mairiang E, Thinkhamrop B, Laha T, Kaewkes S, Sithithaworn P, Tessana S, Loukas A, Brindley PJ, Bethony JM. Advanced periductal fibrosis from infection with the carcinogenic human liver fluke Opisthorchis Viverrini correlates with elevated levels of interleukin-6. Hepatology. 2009;50(4):1273–81.
123. Stauffer JK, Scarzello AJ, Jiang Q, Wiltrout RH. Chronic inflammation, immune escape, and oncogenesis in the liver: a unique neighborhood for novel intersections. Hepatology. 2012;56(4):1567–74.
124. Subleski JJ, Hall VL, Back TC, Ortaldo JR, Wiltrout RH. Enhanced antitumor response by divergent modulation of natural killer and natural killer T cells in the liver. Cancer Res. 2006;66(22):11005–12.

125. Tang Y, Kitisin K, Jogunoori W, Li C, Deng CX, Mueller SC, Ressom HW, Rashid A, He AR, Mendelson JS, Jessup JM, Shetty K, Zasloff M, Mishra B, Reddy EP, Johnson L, Mishra L. Progenitor/stem cells give rise to liver cancer due to aberrant TGF-beta and IL-6 signaling. Proc Natl Acad Sci U S A. 2008;105(7):2445–50.
126. Tilg H, Diehl AM. Cytokines in alcoholic and nonalcoholic steatohepatitis. N Engl J Med. 2000;343(20):1467–76.
127. Tsai WC, Hsu PW, Lai TC, Chau GY, Lin CW, Chen CM, Lin CD, Liao YL, Wang JL, Chau YP, Hsu MT, Hsiao M, Huang HD, Tsou AP. MicroRNA-122, a tumor suppressor microRNA that regulates intrahepatic metastasis of hepatocellular carcinoma. Hepatology. 2009;49(5):1571–82.
128. Tsai WC, Hsu SD, Hsu CS, Lai TC, Chen SJ, Shen R, Huang Y, Chen HC, Lee CH, Tsai TF, Hsu MT, Wu JC, Huang HD, Shiao MS, Hsiao M, Tsou AP. MicroRNA-122 plays a critical role in liver homeostasis and hepatocarcinogenesis. J Clin Invest. 2012;122(8):2884–97.
129. Valcourt U, Kowanetz M, Niimi H, Heldin CH, Moustakas A. TGF-beta and the Smad signaling pathway support transcriptomic reprogramming during epithelial-mesenchymal cell transition. Mol Biol Cell. 2005;16(4):1987–2002.
130. Wan S, Kuo N, Kryczek I, Zou W, Welling TH. Myeloid cells in hepatocellular carcinoma. Hepatology. 2015;62(4):1304–12.
131. Wang Z, Li Y, Sarkar FH. Signaling mechanism(s) of reactive oxygen species in epithelial-mesenchymal transition reminiscent of cancer stem cells in tumor progression. Curr Stem Cell Res Ther. 2010;5(1):74–80.
132. Wang Z, Qiu SJ, Ye SL, Tang ZY, Xiao X. Combined IL-12 and GM-CSF gene therapy for murine hepatocellular carcinoma. Cancer Gene Ther. 2001;8(10):751–8.
133. Weaver CT, Harrington LE, Mangan PR, Gavrieli M, Murphy KM. Th17: an effector CD4 T cell lineage with regulatory T cell ties. Immunity. 2006;24(6):677–88.
134. Wei W, Chua MS, Grepper S, So SK. Blockade of Wnt-1 signaling leads to anti-tumor effects in hepatocellular carcinoma cells. Mol Cancer. 2009;8:76.
135. Weng HL, Liu Y, Chen JL, Huang T, Xu LJ, Godoy P, Hu JH, Zhou C, Stickel F, Marx A, Bohle RM, Zimmer V, Lammert F, Mueller S, Gigou M, Samuel D, Mertens PR, Singer MV, Seitz HK, Dooley S. The etiology of liver damage imparts cytokines transforming growth factor beta1 or interleukin-13 as driving forces in fibrogenesis. Hepatology. 2009;50(1):230–43.
136. Wieckowska A, Papouchado BG, Li Z, Lopez R, Zein NN, Feldstein AE. Increased hepatic and circulating interleukin-6 levels in human nonalcoholic steatohepatitis. Am J Gastroenterol. 2008;103(6):1372–9.
137. Wilhelm SM, Adnane L, Newell P, Villanueva A, Llovet JM, Lynch M. Preclinical overview of sorafenib, a multikinase inhibitor that targets both Raf and VEGF and PDGF receptor tyrosine kinase signaling. Mol Cancer Ther. 2008;7(10):3129–40.
138. Willis BC, Liebler JM, Luby-Phelps K, Nicholson AG, Crandall ED, du Bois RM, Borok Z. Induction of epithelial-mesenchymal transition in alveolar epithelial cells by transforming growth factor-beta1: potential role in idiopathic pulmonary fibrosis. Am J Pathol. 2005;166(5):1321–32.
139. Xu H, He JH, Xiao ZD, Zhang QQ, Chen YQ, Zhou H, Qu LH. Liver-enriched transcription factors regulate microRNA-122 that targets CUTL1 during liver development. Hepatology. 2010;52(4):1431–42.
140. Yamaguchi R, Yano H, Iemura A, Ogasawara S, Haramaki M, Kojiro M. Expression of vascular endothelial growth factor in human hepatocellular carcinoma. Hepatology. 1998;28(1):68–77.
141. Yin M, Wheeler MD, Kono H, Bradford BU, Gallucci RM, Luster MI, Thurman RG. Essential role of tumor necrosis factor alpha in alcohol-induced liver injury in mice. Gastroenterology. 1999;117(4):942–52.
142. Zenewicz LA, Yancopoulos GD, Valenzuela DM, Murphy AJ, Karow M, Flavell RA. Interleukin-22 but not interleukin-17 provides protection to hepatocytes during acute liver inflammation. Immunity. 2007;27(4):647–59.

143. Zhang JP, Yan J, Xu J, Pang XH, Chen MS, Li L, Wu C, Li SP, Zheng L. Increased intratumoral IL-17-producing cells correlate with poor survival in hepatocellular carcinoma patients. J Hepatol. 2009;50(5):980–9.
144. Zhou SL, Dai Z, Zhou ZJ, Wang XY, Yang GH, Wang Z, Huang XW, Fan J, Zhou J. Overexpression of CXCL5 mediates neutrophil infiltration and indicates poor prognosis for hepatocellular carcinoma. Hepatology. 2012;56(6):2242–54.

Index

T.F. Greten (ed.), *Immunotherapy of Hepatocellular Carcinoma*,
DOI 10.1007/978-3-319-64958-0